Handbook of ... matology

For Hazel, my wife, who has sacrificed many hours typing and re-typing the manuscript, when she could have been talking to the children and grandchildren

Handbook of
Paediatric
Dermatology

Julian L Verbov

MD, FRCP, FRCPCH, FIBiol

Professor of Dermatology
Consultant Paediatric Dermatologist
Royal Liverpool Children's Hospital
Alder Hey
Liverpool, UK

MARTIN DUNITZ

© 2000 Martin Dunitz Ltd, a member of the Taylor & Francis group

First published in the United Kingdom in 2000
by Martin Dunitz Ltd, The Livery House, 7–9 Pratt Street, London NW1 0AE

Tel.:   +44 (0) 20 74822202
Fax.:   +44 (0) 20 72670159
E-mail: info@dunitz.co.uk
Website: http://www.dunitz.co.uk

Reprinted in paperback 2002

A CIP record for this book is available from the British Library.

ISBN 1 84184 222 2

Distributed in the USA by
Fulfilment Center
Taylor & Francis
7625 Empire Drive
Florence, KY 41042, USA
Toll Free Tel.: +1 800 634 7064
E-mail: cserve@routledge_ny.com

Distributed in Canada by
Taylor & Francis
74 Rolark Drive
Scarborough, Ontario M1R 4G2, Canada
Toll Free Tel.: +1 877 226 2237
E-mail: tal_fran@istar.ca

Distributed in the rest of the world by
Thomson Publishing Services
Cheriton House
North Way
Andover, Hampshire SP10 5BE, UK
Tel.: +44 (0)1264 332424
E-mail: salesorder.tandf@thomsonpublishingservices.co.uk

Composition by Scribe Design, Gillingham, Kent
Printed and bound in Singapore by Kyodo Printing pte Ltd.

Contents

Acknowledgements

I am very grateful to Mr Dave Adkins, Chief Medical Photographer of the Royal Liverpool University Hospitals Department of Medical Illustration and Mr Tony Hanmer, Chief Medical Photographer of the Royal Liverpool Children's Hospital (Alder Hey) Department of Medical Illustration for providing and allowing reproduction of many of the photographs in the book. I thank parents who always freely gave permission for their children to be photographed. The vast majority of photographs are of my own patients but I sincerely thank colleagues who have permitted me to use photographs of their patients.

JLV

Preface

The aim of this book is to make the diagnosis of childhood skin disorders easier for the reader. Common skin disorders are the most commonly seen and so these have a priority. However, some less common disorders are included because recognition of them is also important.

What conditions do I usually see in a busy routine large children's hospital skin out-patient clinic? Atopic eczema, of course, is the most common disorder seen and is the cause of much misery to infant, child, family and friends. Scalp hair loss, psoriasis, moles (melanocytic naevi), strawberry marks (capillary haemangiomas) and scabies are regularly seen. Viral warts over limbs and molluscum contagiosum are very common but self-limiting and do not need to be seen routinely at a hospital clinic because of the many more important disorders that require a specialist clinic opinion.

The diagnosis of scabies is often missed but this infestation is so important to diagnose – by the time I see the itching child a secondary urticarial and/or eczematized eruption may have appeared with many lesions secondarily infected. Such a complicated picture will obscure the underlying diagnosis (burrows may not be visible) but a careful examination and the history of itching in close contacts is important.

The general public have become much more aware in recent years of the dangers of sun exposure and of the importance of changes in moles (particularly in shape, colour, or size – other than with age) as possible signs of malignant change. The Solar UV Index, which identifies the strength of ultraviolet radiation on a numerical scale of 1 to 20 is now in worldwide use by weather forecasters and is a useful advance in Health Education. Fortunately, the likelihood of malignant change in a mole in the under-14 age group is extremely small.

The newborn, atopic dermatitis, infections, erythemato-squamous eruptions, hair, nails, connective tissue disorders, drug eruptions, inherited disorders, acne, light eruptions, and trauma, are many of the topics covered in this text.

Many diseases mentioned do also occur in adults, but their natural history and management is often different in children. I recognise the divisions: newborn (birth to one month), infancy (one month to two years), childhood (two to 12 years), and adolescence (12 to 16 years), but because so many conditions do occur at any age, I considered it more sensible not to divide the book artificially. However, a chapter on the newborn was essential, but even here some of the conditions mentioned can initially occur at an older age or continue into infancy or childhood, and similarly some conditions only mentioned elsewhere may present in the newborn. Some congenital conditions, such as sebaceous naevi, do not appear in the chapter on the newborn because they are usually first noticed later on. I have tried to reduce overlap to a minimum although a few disorders do merit multiple mention.

I hope that a wide readership will include dermatologists in training, paediatricians, family practitioners, clinical medical officers, senior medical students and nurses. This book largely represents my own experience, which I am pleased to share with the reader. It will be a source of satisfaction to me if this book stimulates further interest in this important branch of dermatology.

Julian L Verbov
Royal Liverpool Children's Hospital
Alder Hey
Liverpool, UK

1
The Newborn

CONTENTS

Genodermatoses
   Ichthyoses
      Sex-linked ichthyosis 1.37
      Collodion baby 1.38–1.39
      Non-bullous ichthyosiform erythroderma 1.40
      Lamellar ichthyosis 1.41
      Epidermolytic hyperkeratosis 1.42–1.44
   Incontinentia pigmenti (Bloch–Sulzberger) 1.45–1.47
   Epidermolysis bullosa
      Simplex
         Dowling–Meara 1.48–1.49
      Dystrophic
         autosomal recessive 1.50–1.51
Neonatal lupus erythematosus 1.52
Langerhans cell histiocytosis (*see also 4.37*) 1.53–1.54
Iatrogenic ulceration 1.55

INTRODUCTION

In this chapter some conditions which may appear in the first month of life are considered. Haemangiomas and other naevi are the conditions most commonly referred to me in this age group. Bullous impetigo and staphylococcal scalded skin syndrome are regularly seen in babies admitted via the Accident and Emergency Department. Minor conditions such as cutis marmorata, milia, cradle cap and salmon patches would generally be recognized by the Health Visitor and usually would not be referred to my clinic.

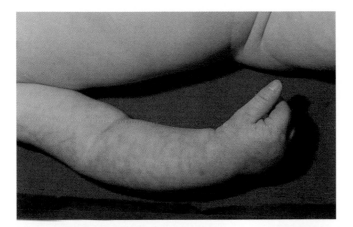

Figure 1.1 Cutis marmorata: prominent over the forearm. This is a normal reticulated bluish mottling of the skin seen on the trunk and extremities. It is a physiological response to chilling with resultant dilatation of capillaries and small venules and unlike *livedo reticularis* (see Chapter 7) disappears with re-warming.

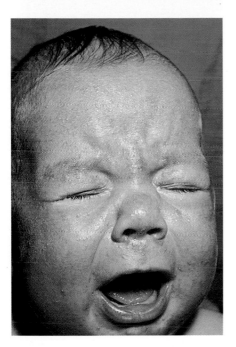

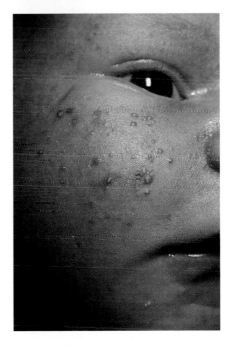

Figure 1.2 Milia: small white papules can be seen over the forehead, cheeks and inferior to the nose. These lesions commonly occur on the face of the newborn and result from retention of keratin and sebaceous material within the pilosebaceous apparatus of the neonate. They appear as multiple pearly white or yellow 1–2 mm papules. These keratin cysts usually rupture on to the skin surface and disappear within a few weeks of birth.

Figure 1.3 Sebaceous gland hyperplasia: a 23-day-old neonate showing florid yellow papules. This is manifested by multiple yellow tiny papules on the nose, cheeks and upper lips of newborn infants. They are a manifestation of maternal androgen stimulation and are a temporary phenomenon resolving in a few weeks. Although sometimes considered the same as milia, the sebaceous hyperplasia papules tend to be more florid and are not cystic.

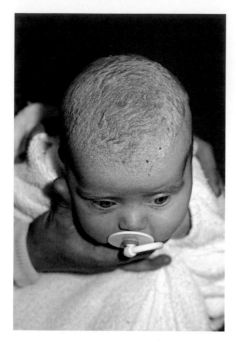

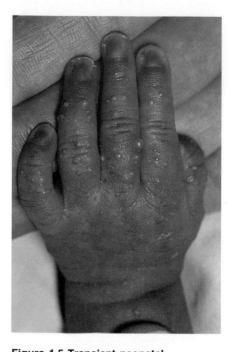

Figure 1.4 Cradle cap: thick scalp scaling is shown but this separated quite easily. Yellowish scalp scaling is common in neonates and infants. It may occur alone or be part of an often widespread flexural eruption, *infantile seborrhoeic dermatitis* (see Chapter 4).

Figure 1.5 Transient neonatal pustulosis: a 2-week-old neonate. This is an uncommon benign self-limiting condition of unknown aetiology in which scanty superficial sterile pustules without associated erythema are present at birth. Neck and trunk are common sites, but lesions can occur anywhere. Individual pustules either disappear spontaneously within a few days, rupture and peel, or dry producing a flat brownish crust which can be gently scratched away. New lesions may continue to appear for a few weeks.

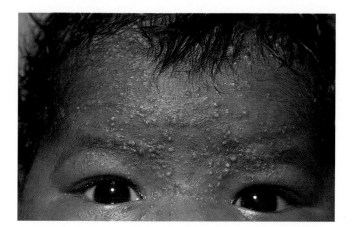

Figure 1.6 Miliaria: forehead lesions showing in a 3-week-old baby. This is caused by eccrine sweat retention and is characterized by an erythematous papulo-vesicular eruption that is distributed particularly over the face, neck, upper chest and back, but anywhere where there is excessive heating of the skin. Therapy is directed towards avoidance of excessive heat and humidity with lightweight loose clothing recommended.

Staphylococcal infections

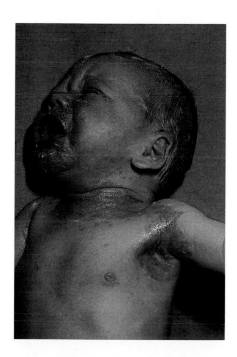

Figure 1.7 Staphylococcal scalded skin syndrome: a 12-day-old child showing facial erythema and perioral, neck and axillary involvement. SSSS presents as a widespread tender erythema which develops within a few hours to a few days, and is worse over the face, neck, axillae and groins. This is followed by the appearance of large flaccid bullae. The upper epidermis peels away leaving scald-like areas. Sometimes the eruption may be more localized as in this neonate and erythema without blistering is also seen. Treatment with a penicillinase-resistant penicillin, fusidic acid, erythromycin or appropriate cephalosporin is indicated for this infection, due to production of an epidermolytic toxin from phage Group 2 benzylpenicillin-resistant staphylococci. Recovery is within 5–7 days. The eruption may be preceded by purulent conjunctivitis or other infection and often there is a history of typical *impetigo* in a sibling (see Chapter 3).

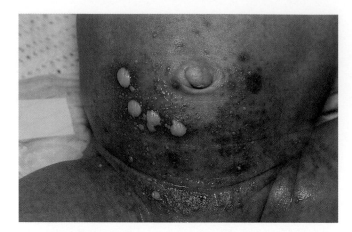

Figure 1.8 Bullous impetigo: a 12-day-old baby with typical bullous lesions containing pus. This is a purely bullous or vesicular form of impetigo seen particularly in the newborn. Treatment is as for staphylococcal scalded skin syndrome.

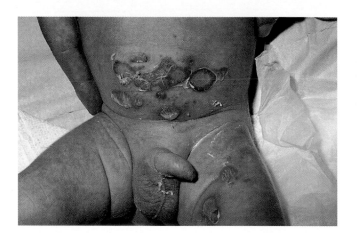

Figure 1.9 Bullous impetigo: another baby, 2 weeks old, showing bullae, some of which show a fluid level of pus. It began at 9 days.

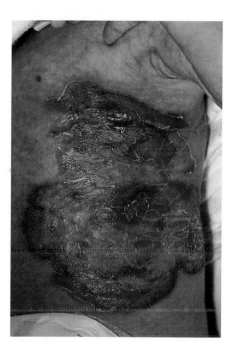

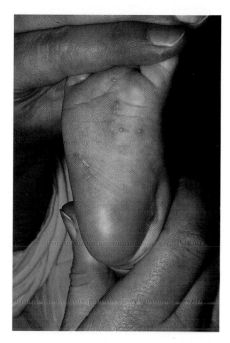

Figure 1.10 Bullous impetigo: a 7-week-old infant. This more diffuse extending bullous lesion over chest and abdomen occurred post-operatively following lung surgery and was associated with skin suture infection.

Figure 1.11 Scabies: burrows are visible in this 2-month-old infant. Scabies must not be forgotten even in the first month of life and other members of the family will usually be itching. If the napkin area is involved papules will be visible and evidence of scabies will be found over the palms, soles and trunk. Treatment is discussed in Chapter 3.

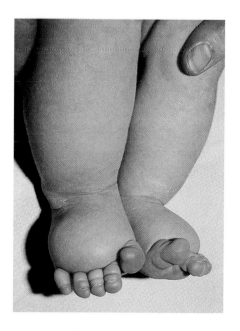

Figure 1.12 Congenital lymphoedema: affecting the lower legs in a 3-week-old male; he gradually improved. Lymphoedema indicates diffuse soft-tissue swelling caused by accumulation of lymph due to inadequate lymphatic drainage. In congenital lymphoedema the area involved is swollen at birth. The swelling is firm and pits on pressure. When occurring in females, and if hypoplastic toenails are present, *Turner's syndrome* should be suspected.

Congenital hair anomalies

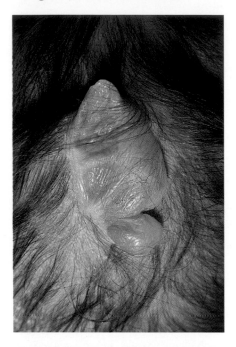

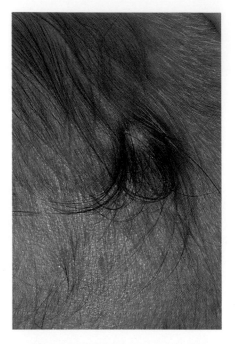

Figure 1.13 Scalp cyst with heterotopic brain tissue: soft, pink, hairless, multilocular lesion – containing clear fluid overlying the left parietal bone and present at birth. This was a solitary lesion and investigations revealed no evidence of any intracranial connection before it was excised uneventfully. This illustrates a rare developmental abnormality to be considered in the differential diagnosis of scalp lesions in neonates.

Figure 1.14 'Hair collar' sign: long black hairs formed a collar around a bald flat round 0.5 cm diameter, clinically superficial, slightly bluish patch over the left parietal region in this 5-month-old infant. Magnetic resonance imaging was normal. This sign can be an indication of heterotopic neural tissue and/or underlying central nervous system malformation.

Disorders of subcutaneous fat

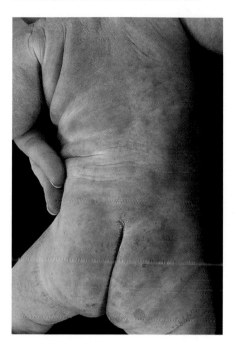

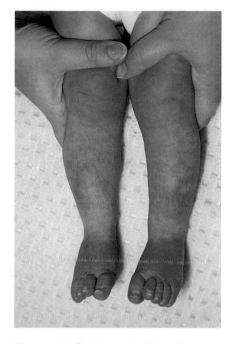

Figure 1.15 Neonatal cold injury: a 3-week-old baby, delivered by Caesarean section. Skin change, particularly over the buttocks, which felt like cold wooden blocks, became visible at 18 days. Indurated skin in folds over the back is also seen. There was no central heating at home. This is a benign self-limiting condition seen occasionally in healthy but often premature newborn babies in the first few weeks of life. Pitting oedema, more marked over limbs, may co-exist with a few sharply-defined woody indurated non-pitting areas of skin feeling cold to the touch. Buttocks and back are favoured areas for the hardened skin but such areas may occur anywhere. Management consists of ensuring that the child is kept adequately warm, and spontaneous resolution leaving no permanent skin change is to be expected within a week or so.

Figure 1.16 Cold panniculitis: affected the legs in a 13-month-old infant who recovered in one week. This condition usually occurs in the newborn and is manifested by warm red indurated nodules appearing after cold exposure. It resolves rapidly although post-inflammatory hyperpigmentation may appear.

Epidermal naevus

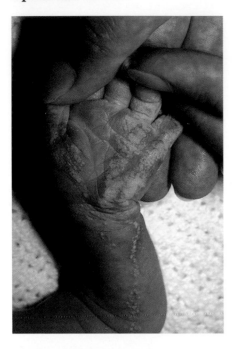

**Figure 1.17 Epidermal naevus –
verrucous type:** palm and forearm in a
neonate with a non-blistering, mainly
unilateral, linear eruption pictured on the
first day of life. Histopathology indicated
an epidermal naevus, a *naevus* being
defined as a malformation of tissue
structures. Such naevi may be localized or
widespread, as in this child. They tend to
grow with the individual, but in this child
the naevus became less prominent during
the first few years of life.

Pigmented naevi

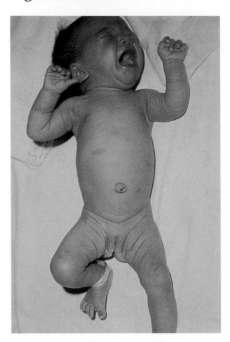

Figure 1.18 Café-au-lait patches: three
of these are visible over the abdomen in a
6-week-old infant. These hyperpigmented
macules with well-defined borders are
usually of no pathological significance
when single. However, before puberty six
or more patches greater than 0.5 cm in
diameter are presumptive evidence of
neurofibromatosis.

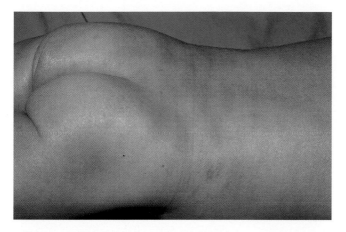

Figure 1.19 Mongolian patches: in a Pakistani infant. These lesions are congenital macular slate-grey or black patches, generally found over the lumbosacral areas and buttocks, but they can occur anywhere on the skin including the face. Most black and oriental babies show them but they are also present in less than 10% of white caucasians. They usually disappear by the end of the first decade. They represent collections of spindle-shaped melanocytes located deep in the dermis. It is important to distinguish them from bruises such as may be seen in non-accidental injury.

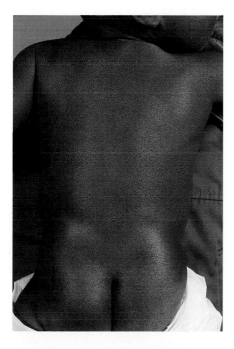

Figure 1.20 Mongolian patches: in a Nigerian infant. Lesions have a blacker appearance in this darker-skinned child.

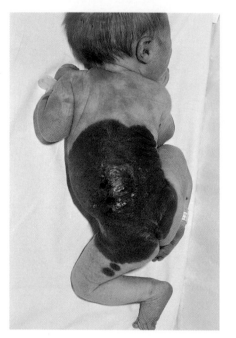

Figure 1.21 Giant pigmented naevus: in a 2-day-old girl. The erosion visible was present at birth and healed within a few days. She is 19 years old now. Histo-pathology of the giant naevus and other smaller ones elsewhere, removed over the years, has always been benign. This is a special form of melanocytic naevus which presents at birth as an extensive (greater than 20 cm in diameter) pigmented hairy area often occupying the lower abdomen and buttocks to cover the napkin area. Such naevi occur less frequently elsewhere. Treatment consists of early surgical excision, if possible, because of the 6% risk of malignant change in such lesions: malignant change (to malignant melanoma) most commonly occurs during the first decade and regular follow-up is essential.

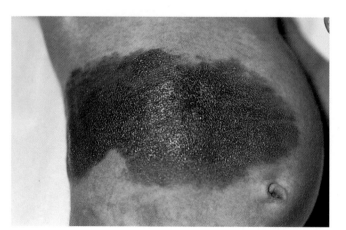

Figure 1.22 Giant pigmented naevus: over the right side of the trunk.

Vascular naevi

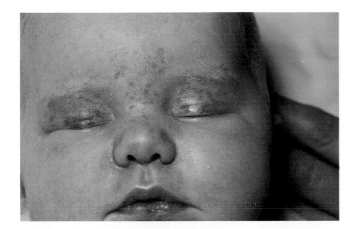

Figure 1.23 Salmon patch: striking lesions over eyelids. This is a common congenital pink area with distended capillaries situated over the forehead, glabella, upper eyelids, nape of neck and lumbosacral region. No treatment is necessary because facial lesions tend to fade in the first year of life but nuchal and lumbosacral lesions tend to persist; the nuchal lesion usually becomes covered by hair and thus becomes unnoticed in time.

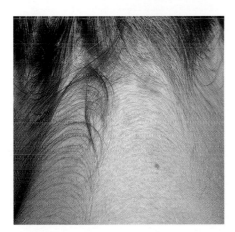

Figure 1.24 Salmon patch: a common site over the nape of the neck (so-called stork bite).

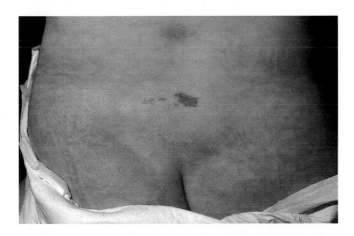

Figure 1.25 Salmon patch: a not unusual site over lower back in a 8-month-old infant.

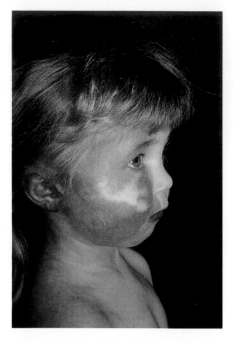

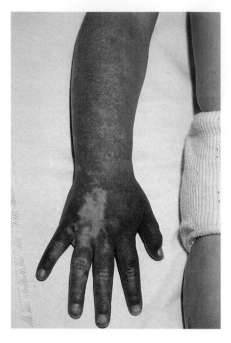

Figure 1.26 Port-wine stain (naevus flammeus)**:** extensive lesion on the face in a 2½-year-old child. This is a vascular malformation, present at birth and is composed of irregularly dilated endothelial-lined capillary vessels confined to the upper dermis; no proliferation of endothelial cells is seen. They do not involute although some fade in colour. They may occur at any skin site and there may be adjacent mucosal involvement. However, they are most common over the head and neck. An association of facial port-wine stain with congenital glaucoma should be appreciated particularly as the glaucoma is usually asymptomatic early in life. Laser therapy is available to treat many skin lesions but not all lesions are suitable and cosmetic camouflage remains a useful tool. Port-wine stains involving the supraorbital region are particularly likely to be associated with similar lesions involving the meninges on the same side, constituting the *Sturge–Weber* syndrome. Manifestations of Sturge–Weber syndrome, such as epilepsy and hemiplegia, may appear in the first year of life but would be unusual to present in the neonate.

Figure 1.27 Port-wine stain: note the sparing of part of the back of the hand in this upper-limb stain.

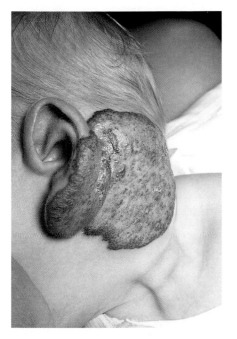

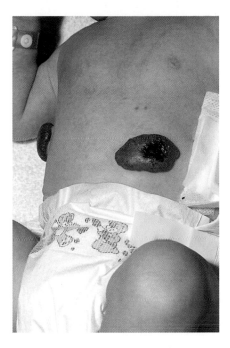

Figure 1.28 Capillary haemangioma
(strawberry mark): a large haemangioma
both behind and involving the pinna. This
may present at birth but generally appears
in the first month of life. Prematurity is a
predisposing factor in the appearance of
such marks. Common sites are the head,
neck and trunk. They are more common
in females and occur in 10–12% of
infants. They appear as well-defined,
small telangiectatic areas and grow to
raised red lobulated tumours with
capillaries visible over the surface. They
grow rapidly with the child in the first 8–18
months of life and then become
stationary, involuting over the next 5–8
years. Residual scarring may follow the
often frictional lesion, that bleeds slightly,
becomes infected, or ulcerates.
Haemangiomas (capillary, mixed,
cavernous) that grow rapidly, are
destructive, or appear at vital structures
(such as the eyes, larynx, or pharynx)
may merit treatment with short-term
systemic corticosteroid therapy, interferon
alpha, or laser therapy to encourage
involution.

Figure 1.29 Capillary haemangioma: in
a 5-month-old infant. This infant had a few
haemangiomas including an eroded one
visible. Such a complication is not
uncommon and may in fact hasten
eventual resolution. However, recurrent
erosion may necessitate laser therapy.

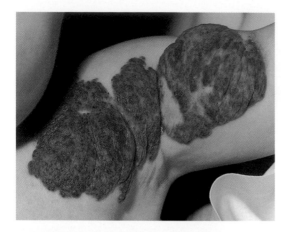

Figure 1.30 Mixed haemangioma: on the left anterior shoulder. This extensive, mainly capillary, lesion also has a deeper (cavernous) element and can be considered a mixed haemangioma. Frequently, a strawberry mark has a deeper (cavernous) element where there are larger mature vascular elements involving both dermis and subcutaneous tissue. These lesions also resolve but resolution may be incomplete.

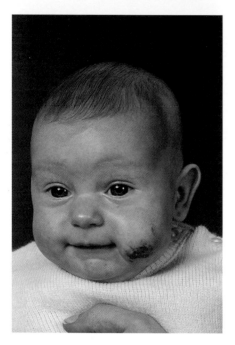

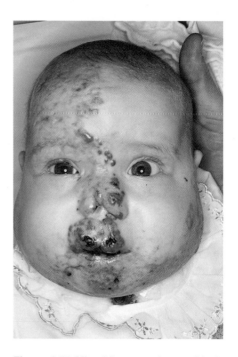

Figure 1.31 Mixed haemangioma: there is a marked subcutaneous (cavernous) element in the lesion in this 3-month-old child. One should note that purely cavernous haemangiomas do also occur, appearing as bluish or bluish-red areas with indistinct borders.

Figure 1.32 Mixed haemangioma: this 6-month-old infant had an extensive facial haemangioma that was destructive over the mid-line: short-term corticosteroid therapy initially and laser therapy (from 2 months old) was helpful. She also had an extensive cavernous haemangioma over the mid-line of the upper chest, and a subglottic haemangioma requiring a tracheostomy until 5 years old. She has improved remarkably with age but will later require plastic surgery to re-fashion her nose and lip.

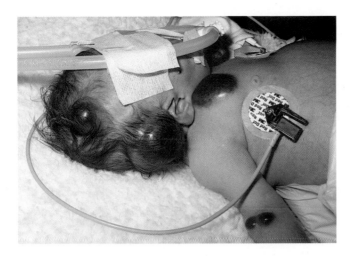

Figure 1.33 Diffuse neonatal haemangiomatosis: a 1-month-old child who showed large solid haemangiomas and who died of complications at 2 months. This is a rare condition, with poor prognosis, in which multiple haemangiomas with multisystem involvement occur. Visceral haemangiomas may involve any organ. The mortality rate is high and death usually occurs as a result of congestive cardiac failure, gastrointestinal bleeding or central nervous system haemorrhage.

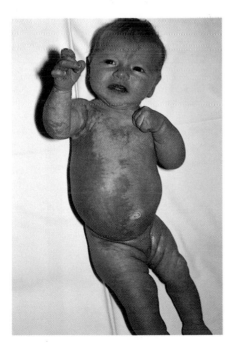

Figure 1.34 Klippel–Trenaunay syndrome: a 5-week-old girl with an extensive port-wine stain over the trunk and enlarged right lower limb. This rare syndrome describes the combination of a port-wine stain with soft tissue overgrowth on a limb with or without bony overgrowth. Port-wine stain is not always present but other vascular abnormalities may be found.

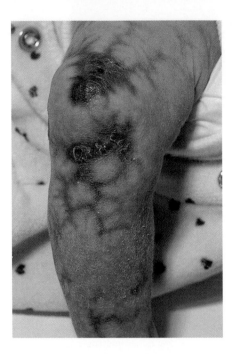

Figure 1.35 Reticulate vascular naevus (cutis marmorata telangiectatica congenita): showing the affected lower limb in a 15-day-old baby. This uncommon combined capillary and venous vascular malformation presents at birth with a flat or depressed reticulate erythema producing a guttering effect. It can occur anywhere but the limbs or trunk are the most common sites. Involvement may be roughly unilateral. Any erosions tend to heal quickly. Spontaneous improvement usually occurs over a period of years. Cutis marmorata (Figure 1.1), which is a physiological response to cold, is unrelated to this condition.

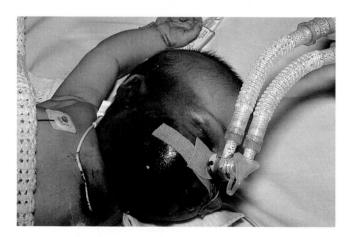

Figure 1.36 Kasabach–Merritt syndrome: an 8-week-old baby who developed respiratory obstruction due to swelling resulting from lesional bleeding. He required interferon therapy and repeated embolization of his lesion. In this syndrome of purpura, thrombocytopenia, disseminated intravascular coagulation and vascular anomaly, it is now considered that the underlying anomaly is not a classical haemangioma but histopathology is of a vascular tumour such as tufted angioma or Kaposiform haemangioendothelioma with lymphatic malformation usually present also.

Genodermatoses

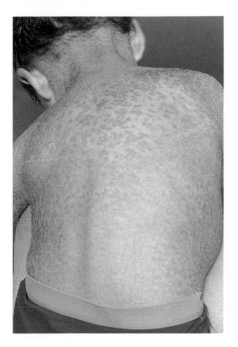

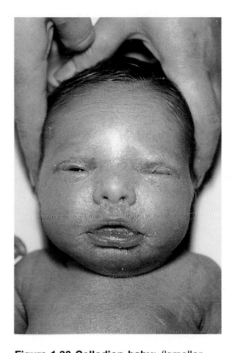

Figure 1.37 Sex-linked ichthyosis: a 2-year-old boy with dark scales over the back and back of the neck. X-linked (recessive) ichthyosis is less common but more severe than the later onset ichthyosis vulgaris. The scales tend to be much larger, polygonal and have a dirty-brown or black colour. The scaliness is frequently obvious at birth. The entire skin surface, including flexures and scalp, may be affected but if the face is involved it is usually only the sides, and increased palm and sole markings are not a feature. The condition is persistent. Steroid sulphatase deficiency is associated with this disorder and its absence permits identification of maternal carriers. Urea-containing emollient and ordinary emollients are helpful.

Figure 1.38 Collodion baby: (lamellar desquamation of the newborn): a female collodion baby at 4 days who had underlying non-bullous ichthyosiform erythroderma. Collodion baby describes an appearance rather than a specific disease. These babies are born enveloped in a shiny transparent but fairly rigid membrane which cracks and peels off after a few days although it may re-form and after peeling the true skin appearance of the child can be visualized. Some form of ichthyosis is usually underlying such as non-bullous ichthyosiform erythroderma, lamellar ichthyosis, X-linked ichthyosis, or ichthyosis vulgaris.

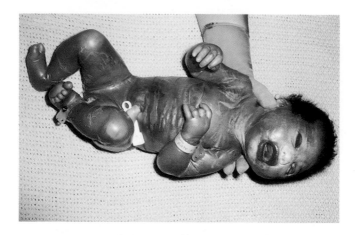

Figure 1.39 Collodion baby: a 1-day-old girl with typical appearance who had underlying lamellar ichthyosis.

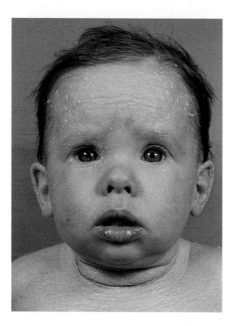

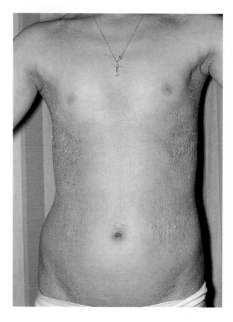

Figure 1.40 Non-bullous ichthyosiform erythroderma: the same girl as pictured in Figure 1.38 at 9 months, showing fine white scaling and faintly red skin. Many years on, her skin remains dry, faintly red and the scalp shows marked scaling. NBIE is an autosomal recessive disorder which may present as collodion baby. The entire skin is dull red with fine white scales superimposed on the erythema. There may be ectropion. Most patients survive and improve showing faint erythema, scaling and hyperkeratosis, most marked over palms and soles, as time goes on.

Figure 1.41 Lamellar ichthyosis: the same girl as pictured in Figure 1.39 at 8 years. She has never had treatment other than emollients. She had scalp scaling and scaling over her trunk. This is a generally more severe but less common form of autosomal recessive ichthyosis than NBIE. Affected skin tends to be less red than in NBIE. Large greyish-brown scales with raised edges occur. Emollients are usually the only therapy required but, as in NBIE, oral synthetic retinoid therapy does have a place in severe debilitating disease.

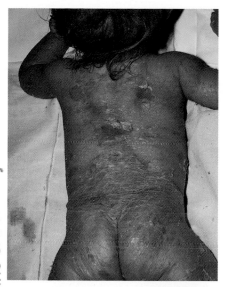

Figure 1.42 Epidermolytic hyperkeratosis (bullous ichthyosiform erythroderma): a 1-year-old girl with superficially eroded skin since birth. This is a rare autosomal dominant disorder in which areas of epidermis peel away shortly after birth leaving raw areas and the appearance may suggest epidermolysis bullosa. The next stage is of crops of bullae which burst to leave raw areas that heal rapidly but have a tendency to become secondarily infected. The background skin is erythematous. In time, warty hyperkeratosis becomes more prominent, appearing strikingly linear in the flexures. Careful handling of the skin, emollients, antiseptic dressings and antibiotic therapy when necessary, will be required. The condition can be diagnosed prenatally by fetoscopy and fetal skin biopsy.

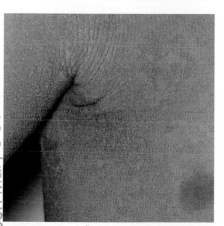

Figure 1.43 Epidermolytic hyperkeratosis: a boy aged 4½ years showing patterned hyperkeratotic lesions.

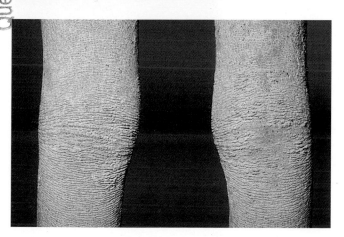

Figure 1.44 Epidermolytic hyperkeratosis: the same boy pictured in Figure 1.43 at age of 13 years, showing typical regular warty hyperkeratosis. He showed some improvement with oral retinoid therapy but this had to be discontinued when he found that blistering was induced. He relied on emollients.

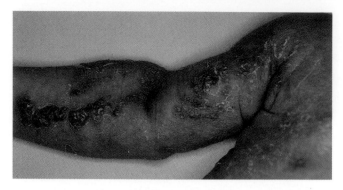

Figure 1.45 Incontinentia pigmenti (Bloch–Sulzberger syndrome): an 11-day-old female with linear blistering. This is an X-linked dominant ectodermal dysplasia which usually presents within a few days of birth generally being prenatally lethal in males. Linear or grouped vesicles appear on the trunk and limbs but by the end of the first month blistering disappears and is usually followed by the appearance of small firm papules and warty plaques. The papules in turn involute leaving angulated and streaked pigmentation and hypopigmentation may also be visible. The condition is variably associated with dental, skeletal, eye and central nervous system abnormalities which must be looked for. Thus a multidisciplinary approach is indicated.

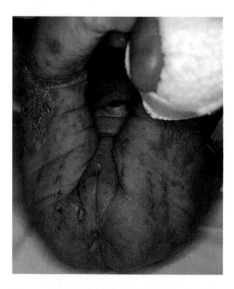

Figure 1.46 Incontinentia pigmenti: the same child pictured in Figure 1.45 showing blistering elsewhere in a typically striking distribution

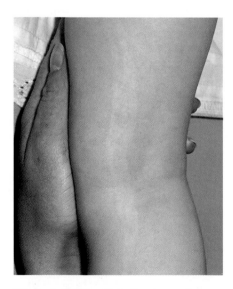

Figure 1.47 Incontinentia pigmenti: a female aged 2 years showing linear hypopigmentation over the lower limb. However, such hypopigmentation does not necessarily occur at sites of previous blisters or warty lesions.

Epidermolysis bullosa

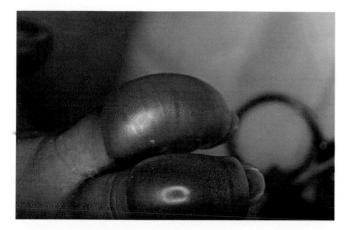

Figure 1.48 Epidermolysis bullosa simplex (Dowling–Meara type): a 3-day-old male with blisters over the fingers. Epidermolysis bullosa indicates a group of inherited non-inflammatory disorders in which blisters and erosions occur with mechanical, often minor, trauma. Epidermolysis bullosa simplex is inherited as an autosomal dominant condition. Onset is usually within the first few months of life. Blisters, which are formed by disintegration of basal and suprabasal cells vary in size and rapidly become tense with clear fluid. The condition tends to be worse in warm weather. Mucous membranes are rarely affected. Healing without scarring is usual. Improvement often occurs with increasing age and protection of the skin from mechanical trauma is paramount in management.

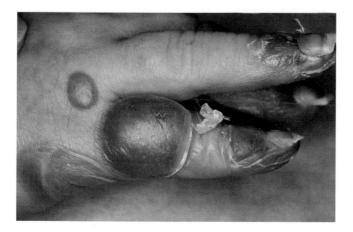

Figure 1.49 Epidermolysis bullosa simplex (Dowling–Meara type): the same boy as pictured in Figure 1.48 at 19 days, showing both blisters and healing. He improved in childhood getting herpetiform blisters over the trunk at times, and he also developed thickening of skin over the palms and soles.

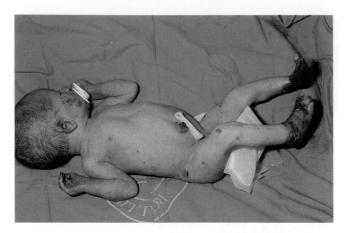

Figure 1.50 Dystrophic epidermolysis bullosa: a boy with this autosomal recessive blistering disease at 3-days old. He is now 5 years old and has retarded physical development, scarred hands and feet following recurrent blistering and mouth and oesophageal involvement. He has a gastrostomy to maintain adequate nutrition. Autosomal recessive forms of dystrophic epidermolysis bullosa are generally severe scarring forms which usually appear at birth, with minor trauma producing blistering and separation of epidermis. Mucous membranes are affected, mouth blisters and erosions being common. Pharyngeal and oesophageal involvement may produce strictures. This is a severe crippling form of disease and genetic counselling and specialist nursing should be available to parents of such children. There are also recessive severe *junctional* forms of epidermolysis bullosa.

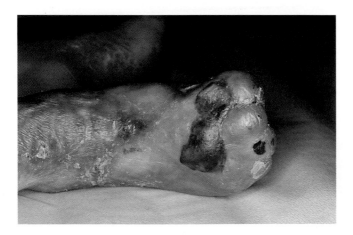

Figure 1.51 Dystrophic epidermolysis bullosa: foot of a female infant with autosomal recessive disease showing marked deformity due to scarring.

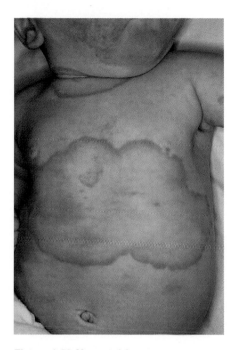

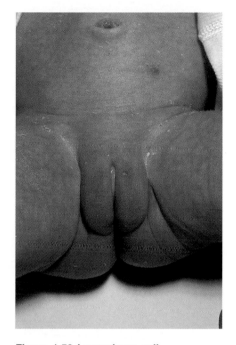

Figure 1.52 Neonatal lupus erythematosus: a 10-week-old male with striking annular erythematous lesions visible. In this rare condition, discoid scaling erythematous lesions occur particularly. There is an associated increased incidence of congenital heart block. Both mother and child are usually positive for the anti-RO/SSA antibody and generally show a speckled pattern of fluorescent antinuclear antibodies. The mother may not show any clinical evidence of systemic lupus erythematosus but may develop it later. Neonates with lupus erythematosus do have an increased risk of developing the systemic disease when older, although lesions resolve and serological markers are usually lost within the first year of life.

Figure 1.53 Langerhans cell histiocytosis: this baby was noticed to have a vesico-pustule on a heel at birth and then developed a few other sterile pustules elsewhere the following week. Lesions are visible over the vulva and abdomen. This is a disorder of unknown aetiology. It can affect single or many organs. Treatment depends on the extent and severity of the disease. Patients with single-system bone or skin disease have a good prognosis and do not usually require treatment. If there is multi-system involvement systemic chemotherapy may be required.

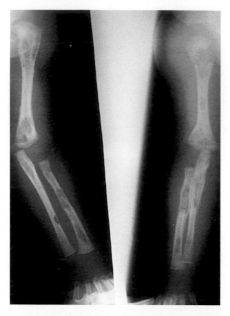

Figure 1.54 Langerhans cell histiocytosis: a radiograph of the same infant pictured in Figure 1.53, showing well-defined osteolytic areas in the limbs. Radiographs were taken because 6–7 weeks after first being seen she was in much pain when lifted and was found to have multiple skeletal lesions and subsequent fractures. She did well following chemotherapy.

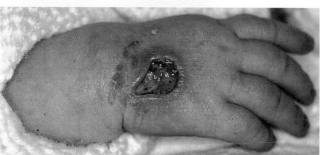

Figure 1.55 Iatrogenic ulceration dorsum hand: in a 27-day-old male. This followed extravasation of intravenous 25% dextrose solution required urgently for hypoglycaemia. It healed with scar formation.

FURTHER READING

Drolet BA, Esterly NB, Frieden IJ. Hemangiomas in children. *N Engl J Med* 1999; **341**: 173–81.

Eady RAJ. Epidermolysis bullosa. In: Champion RH, Burton JL, Burns DA, Breathnach SM, eds. *Textbook of Dermatology*, Vol 3, 6th edn. Oxford: Blackwell Science, 1998: 1817–44.

Hoeger PH, Harper JI. Neonatal erythroderma: differential diagnosis and management of the 'red baby'. *Arch Dis Child* 1998; **79**: 186–91.

Landau M, Krafchik BR. The diagnostic value of café-au-lait macules. *J Am Acad Dermatol* 1999; **40**: 877–90.

Siegfried EC. Neonatal skin and skin care. *Dermatol Clin* 1998; **16**: 437–46.

Van Praag MCG, Van Rooij RWG, Folkers E, *et al.* Diagnosis and treatment of pustular disorders in the neonate. *Pediatr Dermatol* 1997; **14**: 131–43.

Verbov J. Common skin conditions. *Semin Neonatol* 2000; **5**: in press.

2

Atopic and other dermatitis

CONTENTS

INTRODUCTION

The term 'atopy' indicates an inherited tendency to develop one or more of a related group of conditions (asthma, eczema of atopic type, allergic rhinitis, acute urticaria of allergic type) subject to much environmental influence. Atopic dermatitis is the most common skin condition referred to my paediatric clinics and is a source of much misery to affected individuals and relatives. Control of the itching is of prime importance in management.

Atopic dermatitis

Atopic dermatitis (Figures 2.1–2.29) normally appears in the first year of life but uncommonly before 2 months of age. It often affects the face and scalp initially, then extensor aspects of the limbs and later flexures and frictional areas. The face tends to be pale. Atopic skin is often dry and such dryness may sometimes indicate autosomal dominant ichthyosis vulgaris (see Chapter 9), a common association with atopic dermatitis. Atopic eczema, like any eczema, is recognized by pimples (papules) and blisters (vesicles) on a red (erythematous) background, but as the condition is so irritant papules and vesicles are often not easily visible because of inevitable rubbing and scratching which produce excoriations and encourage secondary infection (impetiginization). The prevalence of atopic dermatitis in children up to the age of 12 years in different countries is 12–26% but it should be emphasized that atopic dermatitis may vary in severity from being very mild to very severe. About 60% of affected individuals will clear by the age of 12 and 75% by the age of 16. However some of those who clear will flare again in adult life and prevalence in adults is put at 2–10%. Like asthma, the incidence of atopic dermatitis is sadly increasing and we are uncertain why.

Atopic dermatitis is an inherited disorder with environmental factors very important and abnormal immune function relevant also. *Staphylococcus aureus* abounds on the skin of affected patients. This organism (and streptococci) produces superantigenic toxins which are potent immunostimulatory molecules leading to exacerbation of eczema.

The routine management of atopic eczema involves liberal use of emollients and of preparations containing coal tar, topical corticosteroids, antiseptics, dressings, oral antihistamines (in a dosage that controls the itching) and antibiotics. Applying medications correctly is important and topical steroids must not be abused: topical steroids applied should generally be of mild or moderate potency. Dressings include ointment-impregnated bandages and wet wraps. In wet-wrapping, emollient-diluted steroid is applied to the skin which is then covered with a moistened elasticated stockinette.

The importance of diet must not be overemphasized although breast feeding, which may delay eczema onset, is to be encouraged. Allergic reactions to foods occur in up to 6% of infants. If cows milk intolerance (which includes allergy) is suspected in an intractable eczema, 4–6 weeks off cow's milk (substituting a hydrolysate formula, for instance) may be tried. A dietician should always be involved in any special diets.

In young children, prick testing and blood tests for allergy are unreliable, and are neither useful nor indicated.

It should be noted that contact, as in kissing or bathing, by atopic eczema individuals with sufferers from herpes with active cold sores, must be avoided, because the individual with eczema may acquire eczema herpeticum and can become very ill (eczema herpeticum is usually a manifestation of primary herpes infection).

Atopic dermatitis

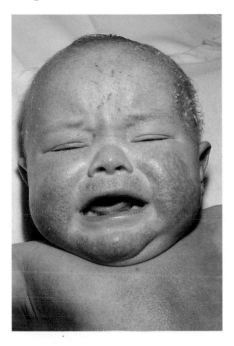

Figure 2.1 Atopic dermatitis: a 5-month-old boy with excoriated atopic eczema. Note the scratch marks over the forehead, the red skin and chapped appearance over the cheeks.

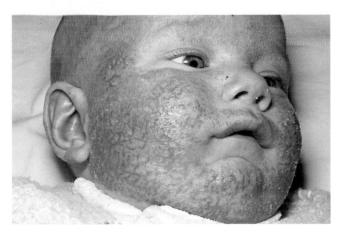

Figure 2.2 Atopic dermatitis: an infant male with dry, chapped eczema over the face.

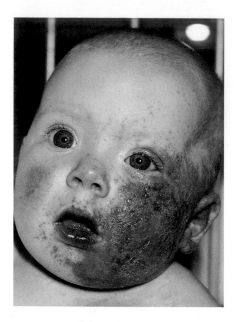

Figure 2.3 Atopic dermatitis: a 6-month-old female with mainly unilateral facial eczema. A day or so later the right side of her face also flared.

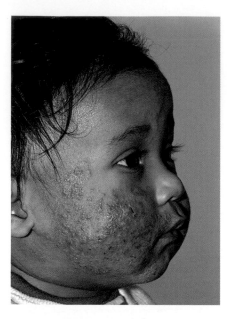

Figure 2.4 Atopic dermatitis: a Sudanese infant boy with facial eczema.

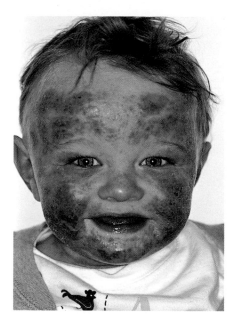

Figure 2.5 Atopic dermatitis: a 1-year-old boy with severe facial eczema. Other affected body areas cleared rapidly but his face was very slow to respond to therapy.

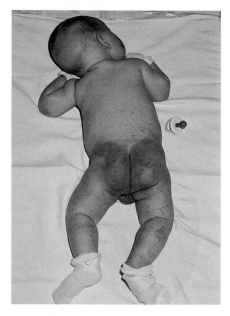

Figure 2.6 Atopic dermatitis: this 5-month-old boy with both atopic and irritant eczema over the buttocks had typical facial eczema also.

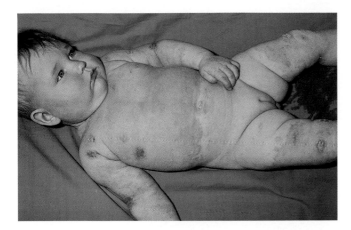

Figure 2.7 Atopic dermatitis: widespread eczema sparing the napkin area, a not uncommon finding.

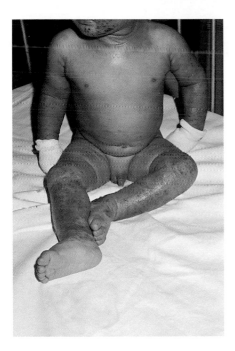

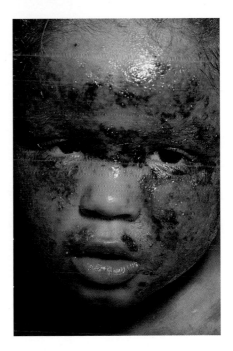

Figure 2.8 Atopic dermatitis: an 11-months-old Egyptian child showing extensor lower limb involvement.

Figure 2.9 Atopic dermatitis: a 4-year-old boy with infected exudative and excoriated eczema. This illustrates well how itchy this condition can be. Oral antibiotics are an essential part of therapy when infection is severe.

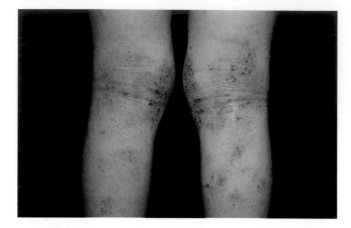

Figure 2.10 Atopic dermatitis: excoriated eczema affecting popliteal fossae.

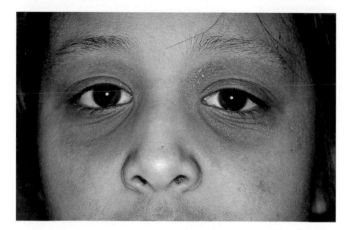

Figure 2.11 Atopic dermatitis: this 7-year-old boy shows evidence of rubbed eyelids and rubbing around the eyes. Extra wrinkles caused by inflammation (atopic wrinkles or Dennie–Morgan folds) are visible below the left eye particularly. As this inflammation subsides it leaves the wrinkling.

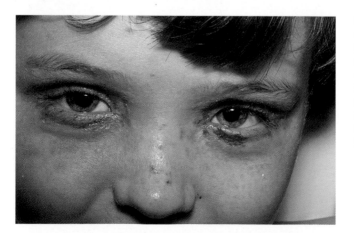

Figure 2.12 Atopic dermatitis: infected, inflamed and excoriated lower eyelids are visible in this boy. This was a recurrent problem over a period of years, requiring frequent hospital admissions.

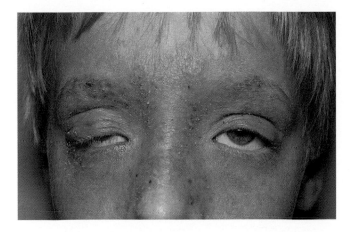

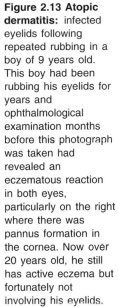

Figure 2.13 Atopic dermatitis: infected eyelids following repeated rubbing in a boy of 9 years old. This boy had been rubbing his eyelids for years and ophthalmological examination months before this photograph was taken had revealed an eczematous reaction in both eyes, particularly on the right where there was pannus formation in the cornea. Now over 20 years old, he still has active eczema but fortunately not involving his eyelids.

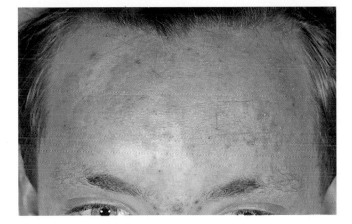

Figure 2.14 Atopic dermatitis: this 13-year-old boy has so rubbed his irritant eyebrow and forehead skin that his eyebrows have been partially (and temporarily) lost.

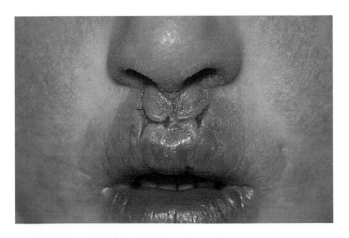

Figure 2.15 Atopic dermatitis: a girl of 4 years old who had been picking and rubbing below her nose for many months (the inflammation gradually resolved with minimal scarring).

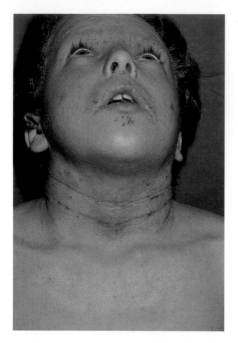

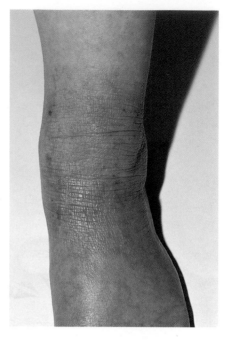

Figure 2.16 Atopic dermatitis: lichenified eczema affecting the neck in a boy of 10 years old. This is a common site and because of it the neck is often held stiffly. *Lichenification* is a peculiar thickening of the skin due to persistent rubbing and scratching which produces accentuation of the skin markings.

Figure 2.17 Atopic dermatitis: lichenification over the ankle in a child with eczema.

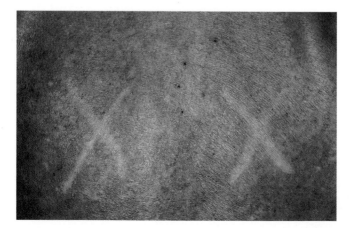

Figure 2.18 Atopic dermatitis: *white dermographism* over the back following gentle stroking of inflamed atopic skin. The small blood vessels in atopic dermatitis show a tendency to vasoconstrict and white dermographism illustrates this. Lesions of white dermographism are flat and not weals (cf. factitious urticaria Figure 8.4)

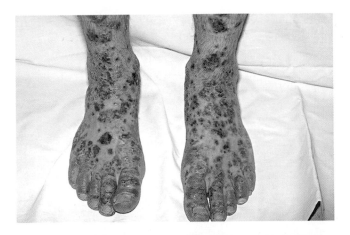

Figure 2.19 Atopic dermatitis: infected excoriated eczema over dorsum feet and lower legs in a 16-year-old boy. Some infected eczema lesions are *nummular (discoid)*. He received an oral antibiotic because bacterial infection is a well-recognized trigger for flare of eczema and should be treated.

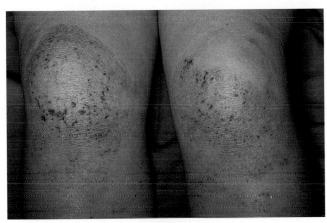

Figure 2.20 Atopic dermatitis: excoriated eczema over the knees in a 3-year-old. Involvement of flexures are more common at this age but this so-called *reverse involvement pattern* is not unusual.

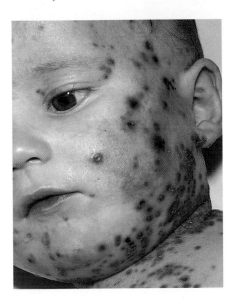

Figure 2.21 Atopic dermatitis: showing primary herpes simplex infection in a 6-month-old atopic child admitted as an emergency – unwell with fever. Lesions are profuse with some umbilicated. He rapidly improved following administration of intravenous aciclovir. The condition is termed *eczema herpeticum* and is not uncommon.

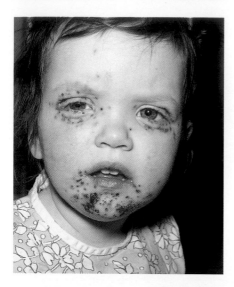

Figure 2.22 Atopic dermatitis: eczema herpeticum over the face in a 2½-year-old. The discrete simplex lesions are secondarily infected.

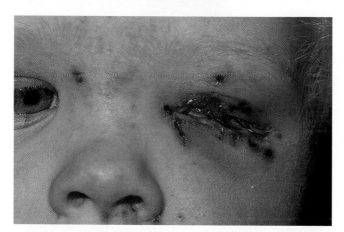

Figure 2.23 Atopic dermatitis: eczema herpeticum with secondary staphylococcal infection affecting the left eyelids in a 2½-year-old atopic child.

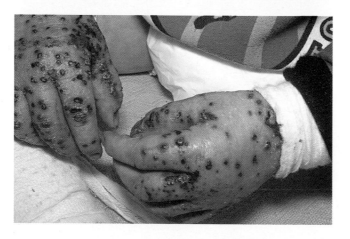

Figure 2.24 Atopic dermatitis: eczema herpeticum involving limbs in a 2½-year-old child.

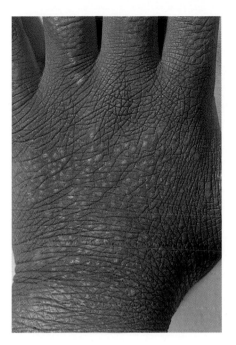

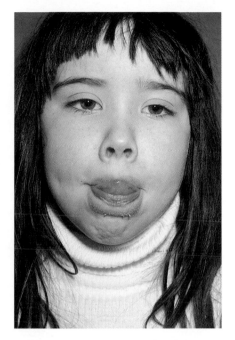

Figure 2.25 Atopic dermatitis: this 4-year-old Somalian child showed eczema papules over the backs of hands and elsewhere over the limbs. *Follicular papules* as part of atopic eczema are common in black children.

Figure 2.26 Atopic dermatitis: showing the effect of *lip licking*. Many lip lickers are atopic, as was this 5-year-old child. Licking the lips makes them drier and the effect of cold in the winter often worsens the problem.

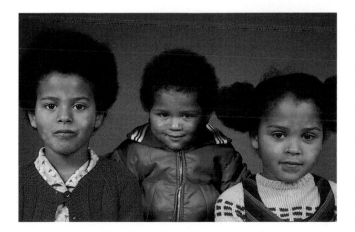

Figure 2.27 Atopic dermatitis: three siblings with *pityriasis alba* over the face. In this entity slight scaling and hypopigmented patches appear particularly over facial skin and it is seen most commonly and more easily in dark-skinned children. Typical atopic eczema may also be present elsewhere but pityriasis alba often occurs alone.

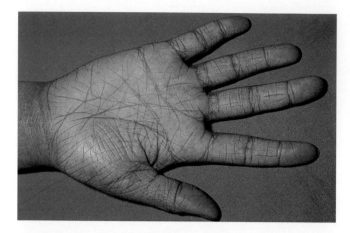

Figure 2.28 Atopic dermatitis: showing *increased palmar markings*. Such markings over the palms and the soles are common both in atopic dermatitis and in ichthyosis vulgaris.

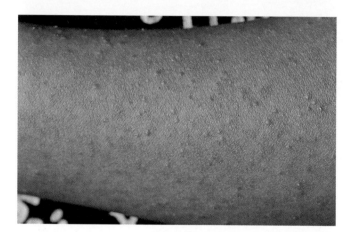

Figure 2.29 Atopic dermatitis: showing *keratosis pilaris* over arm in a 4-year-old child. Such patchy skin roughness, particularly over the backs of upper arms and the front of thighs, due to horny plugging of follicles (keratosis pilaris) is common both in atopic and non-atopic children.

Other dermatitis

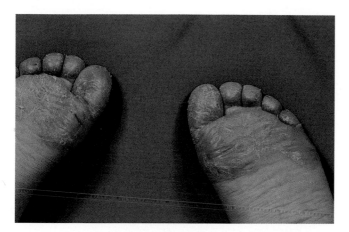

Figure 2.30 Juvenile plantar dermatosis: note the dry peeling skin localized to the forefoot in this atopic boy of 7 years old. This is a frictional dermatitis seen regularly in the 0–17 years group in which itching and burning occur over the plantar aspect of the big toes which then spread to the other toes and the whole forefoot. The affected forefoot becomes red, glazed, dry, cracked, sore and painful and there is often peeling and bleeding. Toe spaces are unaffected. The condition may persist for a number of years. Synthetic footwear with little or absent permeability and poor moisture absorption is an important factor in the aetiology. Atopics are prone to the condition, which also occurs in non-atopics. Cotton socks, leather shoes, urea-containing creams and emollients are recommended.

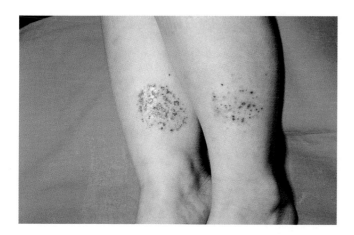

Figure 2.31 Nummular eczema: coin-like patches over the legs of a 2¾-year-old girl. This condition in children is usually a manifestation of atopic dermatitis (see also Figure 2.19). Coin-shaped lesions, which tend to be symmetrical, are seen primarily over the limbs. Secondary bacterial infection of the lesions is common. Nummular eczema has a tendency to be recurrent and chronic.

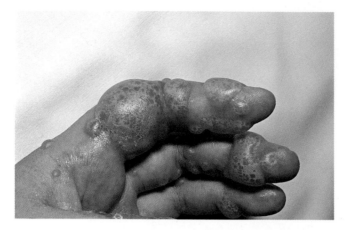

Figure 2.32 Pompholyx (constitutional eczema of pompholyx type): a 12-year-old girl with acute blistering lesions over her fingers. This is a blistering eruption which may be acute or chronic, of unknown cause, affecting the palms, sides of the fingers and the soles. Vesicles may become confluent, forming bullae. Oversweating is present in some cases and the condition used to be called *dyshidrotic eczema*. Onset before the age of 10 is uncommon. Warm weather (as in this child) and emotional stress often seem to precipitate attacks. The child illustrated required a short course of systemic steroids to control the condition, which has not recurred over the past few years.

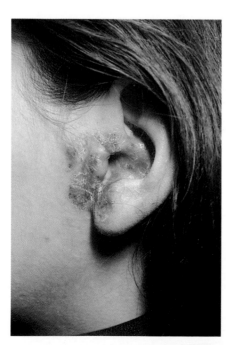

Figure 2.33 Seborrhoeic dermatitis: secondarily infected seborrhoeic dermatitis producing *otitis externa* in a 14-year-old girl. The older child may present with scaling on a background of erythema, between and affecting the eyebrows, over nasolabial folds, involving the ears, and over the trunk. Scalp seborrhoeic dermatitis appears as dandruff. *Blepharitis* may occur in seborrhoeic dermatitis with eyelid margins red and covered with small white scales. Seborrhoeic dermatitis has a susceptibility to become secondarily infected with bacteria and is sometimes referred to as an *infective eczema*. Seborrhoeic dermatitis of this type both in children and in adults is primarily due to a yeast infection (Malassezia ovale).

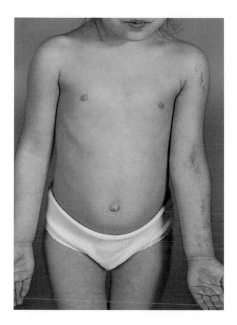

Figure 2.34 Lichen striatus: a girl of 4 years old with a 2 month history of an asymptomatic linear eruption over the left upper limb. The condition is more common in females. This is an uncommon asymptomatic self-limiting, usually unilateral dermatitis of unknown origin, seen in children and young adults. Lichenoid papules appear, usually over a limb and extend in a linear manner over a period of days or weeks. There may be slight scaling associated. Differential diagnosis includes epidermal naevus, psoriasis, and linear lichen planus.

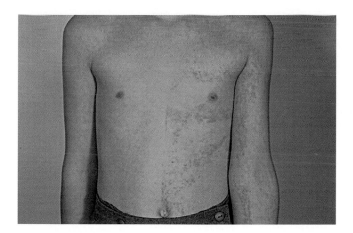

Figure 2.35 Lichen striatus: a girl of 9 years old with eruption over the left side of her trunk and medial left upper limb. It cleared completely in a few months.

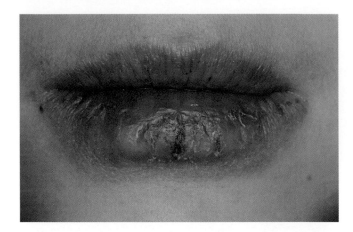

Figure 2.36 Contact dermatitis (irritant type): saxophone cheilitis in a boy of 12. The lower lip dermatitis resulted from contact with the wooden reed mouthpiece. Irritant dermatitis indicates a non-allergic reaction of the skin. The child with *atopic eczema* and *dry skin* is prone to irritant dermatitis.

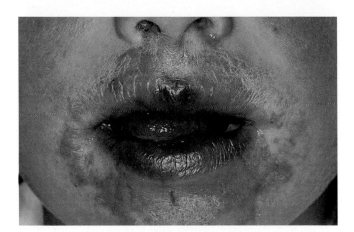

Figure 2.37 Contact dermatitis (irritant type): a 5-year-old lip licker with eczema around the mouth, associated with the use of a dummy at night, rubbing, dribbling, and lip licking.

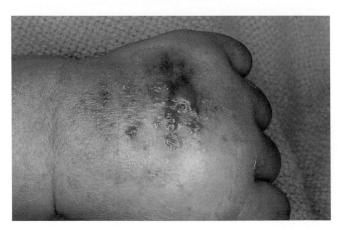

Figure 2.38 Contact dermatitis (irritant type): this 17-week-old male developed acute redness and blistering over the back of his hand due to local anaesthetic gel applied pre-operatively to provide painless venous access. The blistering, which occurred on first exposure to the gel, is uncommon and was considered to be irritant rather than allergic in nature.

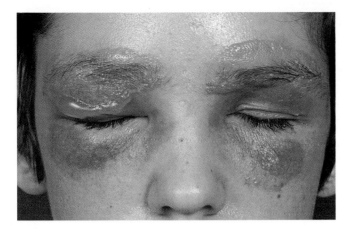

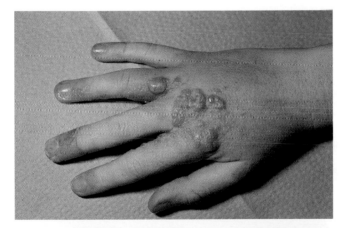

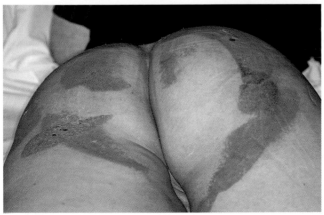

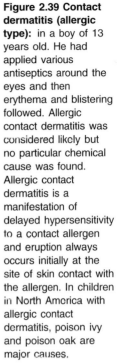

Figure 2.39 Contact dermatitis (allergic type): in a boy of 13 years old. He had applied various antiseptics around the eyes and then erythema and blistering followed. Allergic contact dermatitis was considered likely but no particular chemical cause was found. Allergic contact dermatitis is a manifestation of delayed hypersensitivity to a contact allergen and eruption always occurs initially at the site of skin contact with the allergen. In children in North America with allergic contact dermatitis, poison ivy and poison oak are major causes.

Figure 2.40 Contact dermatitis (allergic type): boy of 10 years old with contact dermatitis (allergic type) over the hand due to adhesive in a plaster. Patch testing revealed him to be allergic to colophony.

Figure 2.41 Contact dermatitis (allergic type): boy of 10 years old who developed a severe contact eruption after application of a hip spica on which the free edges of the plaster of Paris were protected by an adhesive dressing. He showed many positive patch test reactions to adhesives and other chemicals.

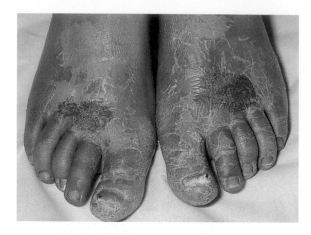

Figure 2.42 Contact dermatitis (photo type): a 12-year-old girl who had tar ointment applied to foot eczema and then exposed her skin to the sun. In photodermatitis some substances are transformed into primary irritants or sensitizers after light exposure and a dermatitis can result. Such reactions may be phototoxic, for example, tars and certain plants such as the Giant Hogweed, or photoallergic as with some perfumes.

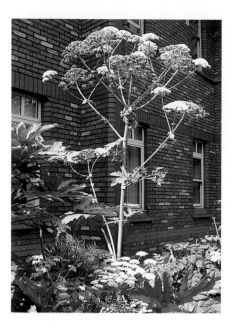

Figure 2.43 Contact dermatitis (phytophoto type): a common cause of phytophoto type dermatitis is the Giant Hogweed plant. The stems are commonly used as peashooters by children, but may provoke a phototoxic reaction due to their photosensitizing furocoumarin content when followed by light exposure. Phototoxic reactions may be sunburn-like or blistering.

FURTHER READING

Brehler R, Hildebrand A, Luger TA. Recent developments in the treatment of atopic eczema *J Am Acad Dermatol* 1997; **36** 983–94.

Charman C. Clinical evidence: Atopic eczema *BMJ* 1999 **318**: 1600–4.

Friedmann PS. Allergy and the skin. II – Contact and atopic eczema *BMJ* 1998; **316**: 1226–29.

Management of atopic dermatitis: current status and future possibilities. In: Hanifin J, ed. *Dermatologic Therapy*, Vol 1, Copenhagen: Munksgaard. 1996.

McFadden J. What is the role of Staphylococcus aureus in atopic eczema? *CME Bull Dermatol* 1999; **2**: 4–6.

McHenry PM. Williams HC, Bingham EA. Management of atopic eczema. *BMJ* 1995; **310**: 843–47.

3

Infections and Infestations

CONTENTS

INTRODUCTION

It is very common for children to present with viral warts, molluscum conta-giosum and scabies and it is important to note that scabies is often unrecog-nized. Thus, if a child is referred with an itchy rash not responding to topical applications, scabies should always be considered especially if other members of the family are itching. Viral warts and molluscum contagiosum are self-limiting and should not be over-treated. Common exanthemata are usually managed by the Family Practitioner.

Bacterial infections

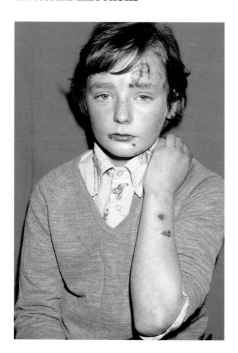

Figure 3.1 Impetigo: facial and forearm lesions in a boy of 11 years old. Impetigo occurs mainly in children, and its occurrence in the newborn as bullous impetigo has been mentioned in Chapter 1. It is usually due to *Staphylococcus aureus* but may be complicated by streptococci. It is often associated with poor hygienic conditions and rapidly spreads among members of the household. Flaccid blisters appear, few or many, most commonly over the face, and these quickly dry and crust. Lesions may also be ringed with a crusted edge. In treatment, removal of crusts is important because bacteria are present in the lesions and infected crusts encourage the spread of impetigo. After removal of crusts, application of antiseptic or antibiotic ointment such as fusidic acid, aureomycin, or mupirocin, is indicated and this may help the occasional complication of acute glomerulonephritis following streptococcal impetigo. More common than impetigo itself is impetiginization of other conditions such as eczema, scabies, head-lice infestation, papular urticaria, and herpes simplex.

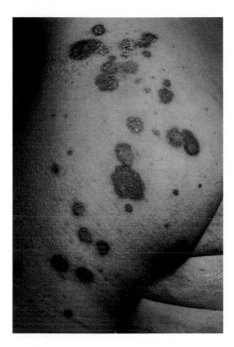

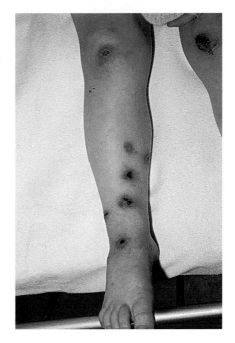

Figure 3.2 Impetigo: an infant of 15 months with impetigo, which was mainly over the buttocks.

Figure 3.3 Ecthyma: a 2½-year-old with leg lesions. Ecthyma is of similar causation to impetigo. Lesions are often multiple and occur over the lower limbs. They have adherent crusts with underlying ulceration.

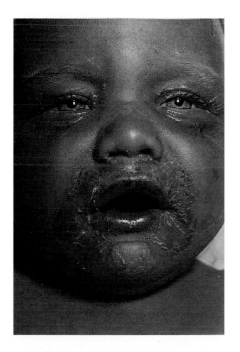

Figure 3.4 Staphylococcal scalded skin syndrome: in a girl of 1 year old. Note crusting around the mouth and eyes and the scalded red skin appearance. This condition is seen usually in the under-five age group and has already been mentioned in Chapter 1. It may be preceded by a purulent conjunctivitis, otitis media, or upper respiratory infection. Staphylococci can be isolated from such foci and there may be a history of skin sepsis in a sibling or other close contact. There may be widespread skin involvement but mucosae are unaffected. Crusted eruption around the mouth is typical. Recovery without scarring is usually within 5–7 days with or without antibiotics, but I treat all cases with systemic antibiotic.

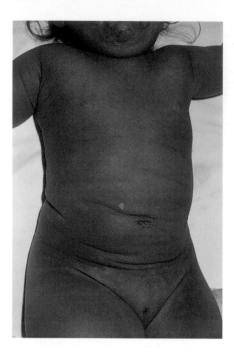

Figure 3.5 Staphylococcal scalded skin syndrome: in the same child as shown in Figure 3.4, showing widespread erythema.

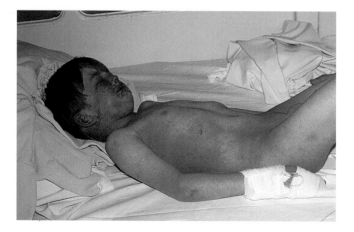

Figure 3.6 Staphylococcal scalded skin syndrome: in a 4¾-year-old boy, admitted as an emergency. Note the scalded skin appearance, facial appearance and raw skin over lower chest.

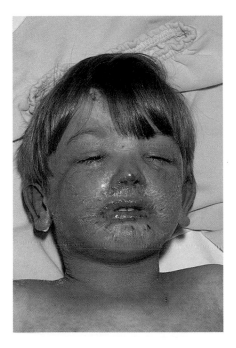

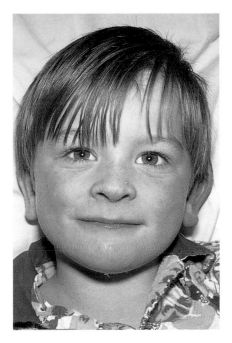

Figure 3.7 Staphylococcal scalded skin syndrome: in the same child as shown in Figure 3.6. Crusting around mouth is striking and typical.

Figure 3.8 Staphylococcal scalded skin syndrome: in the same child in Figures 3.6 and 3.7 showing complete recovery just 4 days later.

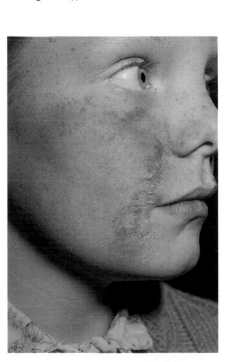

Figure 3.9 Cellulitis: low-grade facial cellulitis in a child. Acute cellulitis (*erysipelas*) is due to Group A haemolytic streptococci entering through a break in the skin usually near the eye, ear, nostril or mouth. Low-grade facial cellulitis is much more common and may be recurrent. Sites of entry are as for erysipelas. When attacks of cellulitis are recurrent there is often an underlying defect of lymph drainage in the affected areas and such patients may show persistent residual lymphoedema associated with tissue fibrosis after recurrent attacks. Although usually due to haemolytic streptococcal infection, cellulitis can be caused by other organisms such as *Staphylococcus aureus*, *Streptococcus pneumoniae*, and *Haemophilus influenzae*.

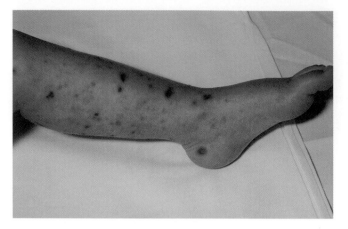

Figure 3.10 Meningococcaemia: purpuric lesions showing
necrosis are visible over the leg. Meningococcal disease is
seen particularly in pre-school children and may present with
purpura, most commonly over the trunk and lower limbs. Fever
and altered consciousness may also be present. In severe
infections, large ecchymoses with sharply-defined borders may
be seen. Lesions result from both intravascular coagulation and
bacterial damage to blood vessels.

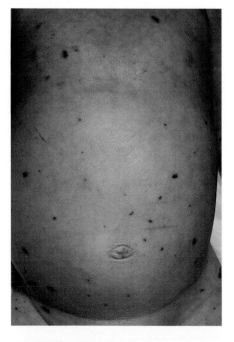

Figure 3.11 Meningococcaemia: purpura
over the trunk in an infant.

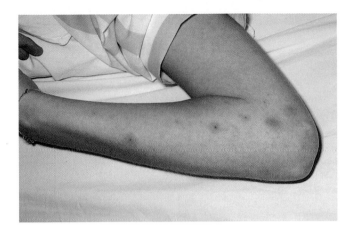

Figure 3.12 Meningococcaemia: girl of 17 years old with scanty purpuric lesions, some with a central papule, over the upper limbs.

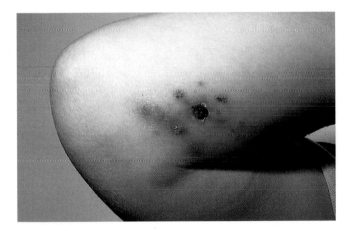

Figure 3.13 Atypical mycobacterial infection: near the right elbow in a 3-year-old girl. Some lesions have broken down and the supratrochlear gland was palpable. No organism was isolated from the excised gland and eruption cleared spontaneously over a period of many months. However, atypical mycobacterial infection seems likely. Abrasions sustained in swimming pools or fish tanks may become infected with atypical mycobacteria such as *Myobacterium marinum*. Most cases present as subcutaneous nodules, ulcers or abscesses at sites of trauma, and the elbows are a common site. Healing usually occurs spontaneously in a few months but antibacterial therapy and/or surgical excision may be required.

Viral infections

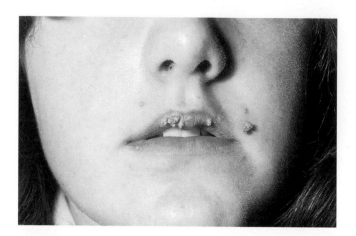

Figure 3.14 Viral warts: lip warts in a girl of 15 years old. Warts are caused by a DNA-containing papillomavirus with many types identified and these infect and replicate in skin and mucosa. Common sites are the hands, feet, knees and face. Virtually all warts disappear spontaneously within three years in children. Warts are uncommon under the age of three years. If plantar warts (verrucae) are painful, the cause is usually overlying callosity, secondary infection or a too-strong application. Reassurance is the best treatment for warts but salicylic acid-containing peeling agents or liquid nitrogen cryotherapy have a place.

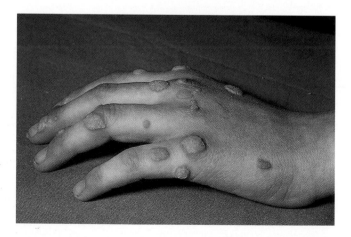

Figure 3.15 Viral warts: florid hand warts in a 7-year-old.

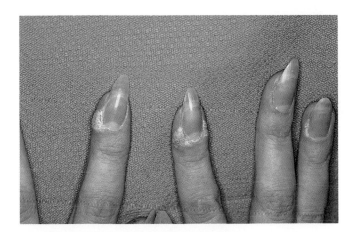

Figure 3.16 Viral warts: nail-fold warts. Warts around finger nails are often associated with spread of the virus by biting and picking at the fingernail folds.

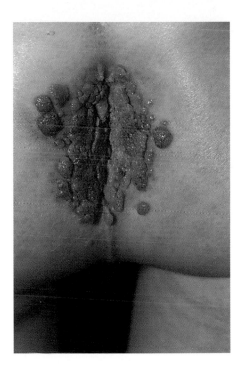

Figure 3.17 Viral warts: florid perianal warts in a 2½-year-old boy. No evidence of sexual abuse was obtained. A complete history of the home environment and contacts is important when genital warts are seen in children but sexual abuse is not commonly found. Topical applications are first-line treatment but surgery, including laser surgery, may be required occasionally.

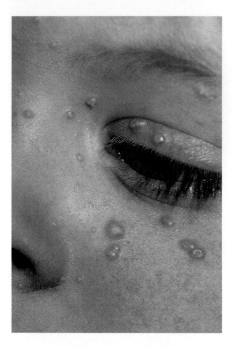

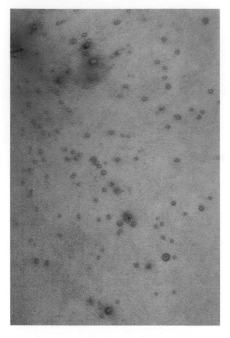

Figure 3.18 Molluscum contagiosum: some of the pearly lesions show umbilication. This is a poxvirus infection common in infants and younger children. Lesions may be single or multiple and appear as discrete pearly papules often with central umbilication. Multiple lesions are common in children with atopic dermatitis and are encouraged by the use of topical steroids. Sometimes localized eczema is visible in an area of mollusca. The trunk, ano-genital region and face are common sites. Lesions tend to disappear spontaneously within one year, often hastened by secondary bacterial infection.

Figure 3.19 Molluscum contagiosum: widespread mollusca in an atopic dermatitis sufferer. Decreased cellular immunity in atopic individuals together with steroid use tend to encourage such skin infection. Note the Köbner phenomenon in one area (see Figure 4.2 also).

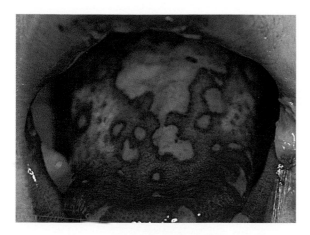

Figure 3.20 Herpes simplex: severe erosive stomatitis in a 5-year-old. This is a primary simplex infection. Primary infection with herpes simplex usually presents as stomatitis between the ages of 1–4 years. It presents as fever with mouth ulceration, often with a few vesicles over the lips, or as a sore throat. The condition usually resolves spontaneously over a period of a week or so, but symptomatic treatment may be required if severe.

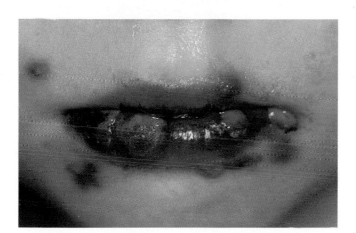

Figure 3.21 Herpes simplex: the same child as shown in Figure 3.20, showing blisters over the lips.

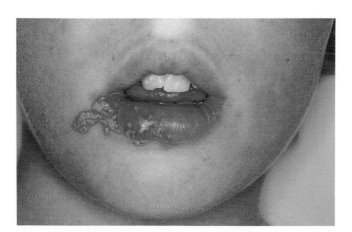

Figure 3.22 Herpes simplex: typical lesions in a boy of 10 years old with secondary simplex infection. The lesions appeared during the course of meningococcal meningitis. Topical aciclovir cream is useful in the treatment of herpes simplex.

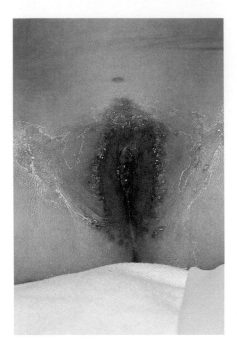

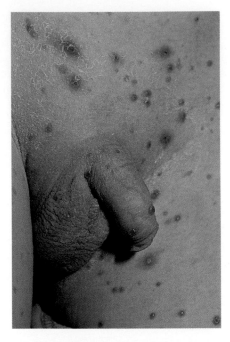

Figure 3.23 Herpes simplex: vulvo-vaginitis due to Type I virus in an 18-month-old infant. She had herpetic stomatitis and transferred infection by touch. She did not but could have acquired the infection by touching someone else's cold sores. The area is reddened and exudative and herpetic lesions are visible at the outer edge of the inflamed skin. History in genital herpes should be thorough to exclude abuse because infection is usually due to Type II virus.

Figure 3.24 Varicella: over the lower abdomen. Eruption appears over the trunk on the second day of the illness and then spreads to the face and limbs. Macules, papules, vesicles and pustules may be seen in any one area at the same time.

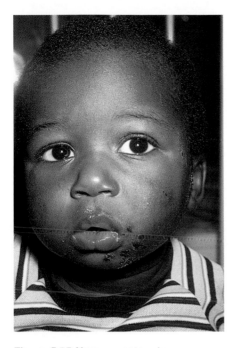

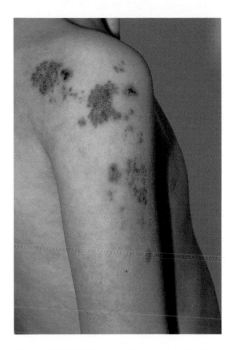

Figure 3.25 Herpes zoster: here affecting the left trigeminal nerve, showing involvement of the left side of the chin, cheek, scalp and anterior to the pinna in a 1-year-old Nigerian infant. His mother had varicella when 8 months pregnant with him and he would have first been exposed to varicella zoster virus at that time. This infection is caused by reactivation of the varicella zoster virus in the individual. The eruption of groups of vesicles on an erythematous background is typically unilateral over one or more dermatomes. Pain, itching or hyperaesthesia in the affected area often precedes eruption by a few days and groups of vesicles may erupt for a few weeks.

Figure 3.26 Herpes zoster: a boy with zoster of C4–C6 distribution over the right upper limb. Symptoms are usually mild in prepubertal children but this boy had much discomfort and received a 10-day course of oral aciclovir.

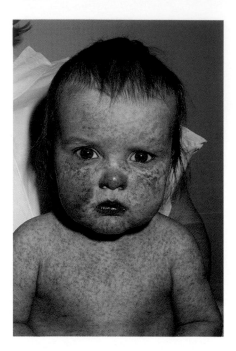

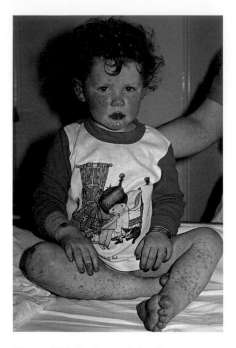

Figure 3.27 Measles: after 3–4 days of the catarrhal stage, Koplik spots on the buccal mucosa disappear while the dark red macular or maculopapular eruption develops. The rash is first seen behind the ears and at the hair line but within hours the whole skin surface becomes affected.

Figure 3.28 Erythema infectiosum: note the slapped-cheek appearance and early maculopapular eruption over the limbs, with the typical perioral sparing. This is due to human parvovirus B19 and small outbreaks of the condition are not uncommon, particularly in the spring. The incubation period is 7–10 days. Red papules on the cheeks become confluent, giving a slapped-cheek appearance and then erythematous maculo-papules appear over the limbs and trunk, and may form a lace-like (reticular) pattern.

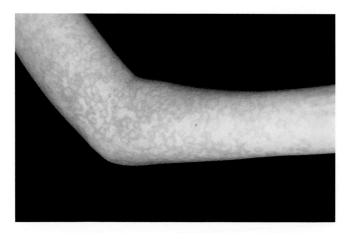

Figure 3.29 Erythema infectiosum: an 8-year-old boy showing lace-like erythema. His twin brother was also affected. The eruption may recur for a few weeks. Like rubella, the parvovirus, B19, can be transmitted transplacentally and the fetus is vulnerable to it.

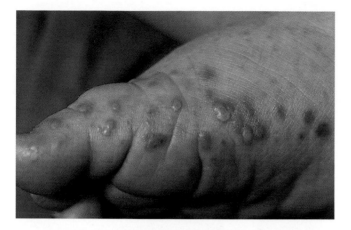

Figure 3.30 Hand, foot and mouth disease: blisters over the foot in a 14-month-old infant. This particularly affects children and is usually due to a Coxsackie virus, or less commonly Enterovirus 71. Usually mild, it presents with a painful stomatitis, with superficial small blisters visible over the buccal mucosa. Similar vesicles occur over the hands and feet and a maculopapular rash may appear over the buttocks. Symptoms persist for about a week.

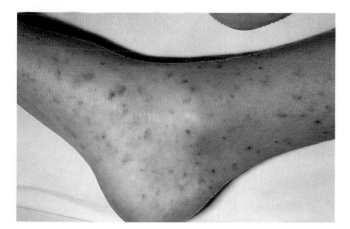

Figure 3.31 Gianotti–Crosti syndrome (papular acrodermatitis of childhood): appearance of red papules over the lower legs followed by malaise and anorexia. Liver enzyme levels were elevated early on in this child. This is a self-limiting skin condition characterized by the sudden onset of coppery–red non-pruritic lichenoid papules over the face, buttocks and extremities, but sparing the trunk. Lesions may look purpuric. Constitutional symptoms are usually mild but there may be anicteric hepatitis, hepatomegaly, and widespread lymphadenopathy. The disorder is probably viral in origin.

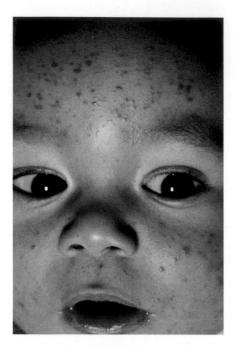

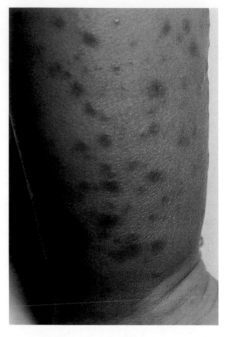

Figure 3.32 Gianotti-Crosti syndrome: a 6-month-old with red papules over the face. He was systemically well.

Figure 3.33 Giannoti-Crosti syndrome: florid papules over the limb in the same child as shown in Figure 3.32.

Fungal infections

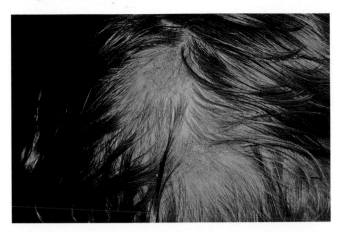

Figure 3.34 Ringworm: two patches of scalp hair loss with little inflammation are visible. Ringworm scalp (*tinea capitis*) was due to *Microsporum canis*. Ringworm infection may affect the hair, skin and nails and infection is acquired from animals (zoophilic), humans (anthropophilic) or from the soil (geophilic). Scalp ringworm (tinea capitis) is common. Ringworm can give rise to markedly inflammatory patches covered with pustules (*kerion*). Scalp ringworm usually manifests as hair loss with visible broken-off hairs with a varying degree of scalp erythema and scaling. In body ringworm (*tinea corporis*) circular lesions are identified by their active, raised, scaling margins. Foot ringworm (tinea pedis) is common and visible toe-space scaling or acute blister formation is seen. Topical antifungals include imidazoles and 6–8 weeks therapy with oral griseofulvin (10 mg/kg body weight daily) is usually effective for scalp ringworm. Ringworm in the over-12 year age group may merit monitored treatment with oral itraconazole or terbinafine.

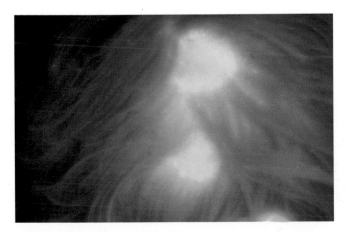

Figure 3.35 Ringworm (tinea capitis): the same child as in Figure 3.34 showing fluorescence of the 2 bald patches under Wood's ultraviolet light. Hairs infected with *M. canis* or *M. audouinii* (an anthropophilic fungus) fluoresce blue/green.

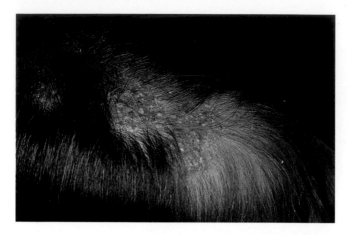

Figure 3.36
Ringworm (tinea capitis): this illustrates hair loss and kerion in a child from North Wales, whose dog also had (*Microsporum canis*) ringworm. The child with a zoophilic infection would not require exclusion from school because infectivity from human to human is only slight.

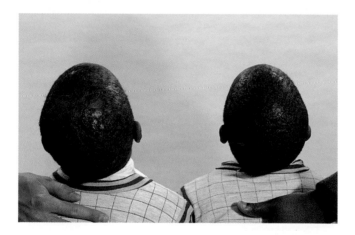

Figure 3.37
Ringworm (tinea capitis): these 6-year-old twin girls from Nigeria began losing hair 4 months after leaving Nigeria. *Trichophyton soudanense* (an anthropophilic fungus) was cultured. The twins were kept off school because of risk of spread to other children and returned after contacts were screened and the twins were non-infective.

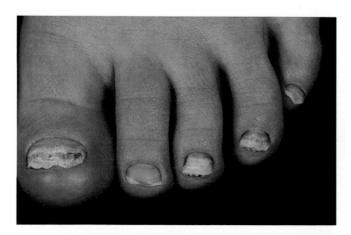

Figure 3.38
Ringworm nails (tinea unguium): a boy of 3½ years old with white, thickened toe nails, abnormal since 8 months old. He probably acquired the infection from a parent with similarly infected toe nails.

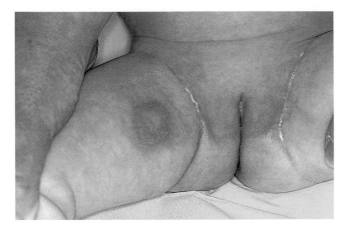

Figure 3.39 Ringworm (tinea corporis): solitary ringed patch over the thigh in 5-month-old showing an inflamed edge. *Trichophyton rubrum* grew from skin scrapings and the lesion responded to an imidazole cream.

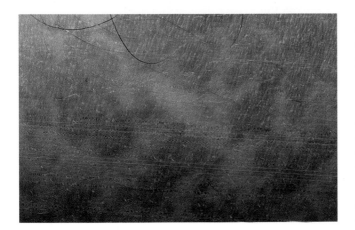

Figure 3.40 Pityriasis versicolor: close-up of brown scaling patches over chest. This superficial fungus infection caused by Malassezia yeasts is most common in young adults but does occur in older children. Scaling patches which may be hypopigmented or hyperpigmented appear. It is usually asymptomatic but it may itch in some individuals. An imidazole cream applied twice daily for three weeks often clears the condition which may recur.

Parasitic infestations

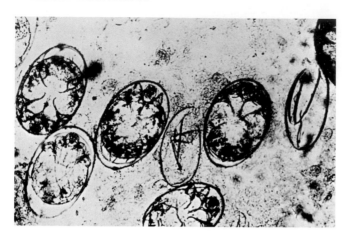

Figure 3.41 Scabies: scraping from a burrow showing numerous larvae and empty egg cases. Human scabies is common and is due to *Sarcoptes scabiei* var. *hominis*. It presents after an incubation period of 2–6 weeks following infestation with the mite, with burrows (the characteristic lesions) over finger and toe spaces, palms, soles, front of the wrists, breasts, axillary folds, buttocks, backs of the elbows and the penis. In infants, who may be only a few weeks old, eruption is often even more widespread, sometimes with papules or nodules over the trunk, and papules, vesicopapules or pustules over the palms and soles. Burrows are not always visible, particularly in hot, humid climates. In scabies, excoriations, eczematized and impetiginized lesions are frequent and a secondary sensitization eruption of urticarial type may complicate infestation. All members of the family, whether symptomatic or not, require treatment. Treatment for this infestation includes an application of permethrin cream (5%) which should be applied over the whole body, including the face if necessary (in infants), and the skin washed thoroughly 8–12 hours later. Malathion (0.5%) in an aqueous base is an alternative preparation to be applied to the whole body including the face if required and washed off after 24 hours: I do not prescribe this in infants less than 6 months old. There is still a place in resistant cases for 25% benzyl benzoate emulsion diluted with 3 parts water in infants, applied below the face to all areas and left on for 12 hours, then re-applied for another 12 hours and finally washed off in the bath. If treatment is carried out correctly at home children do not normally require time off school. Itching in scabies often persists for a few weeks or more, even after successful treatment, and responds to oral antihistamines.

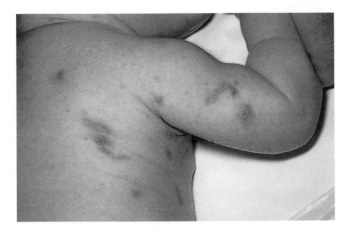

Figure 3.42 Scabies: lesions including burrows in a 2-month-old girl.

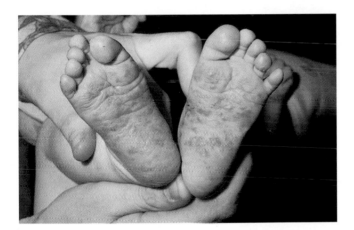

Figure 3.43 Scabies: a 16-week-old infant with multiple sole lesions. In infants, papules, pustules, and vesicles over the soles are common.

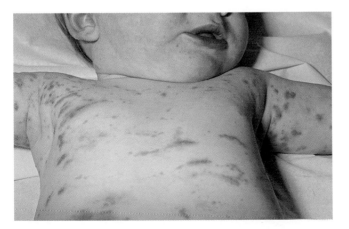

Figure 3.44 Scabies: a 9-month-old baby with urticarial reaction and eczematization of some lesions. He had had scabies for 5 months when seen. Obtaining a history of itching in other family members also, was an important finding even before the infant was examined.

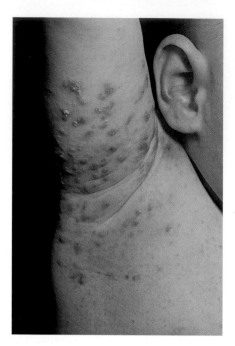

Figure 3.45 Scabies: a 10-month-old infant with florid axillary lesions.

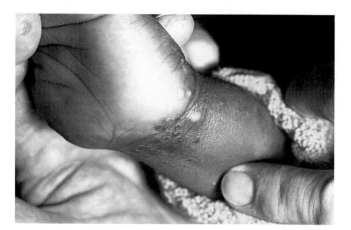

Figure 3.46 Scabies: wrist pustules in a 4-year-old Nigerian child. *Staphylococcus aureus* grew from one of these pustules. The scraping was negative for scabies, but distribution and history of symptomatic family members was important.

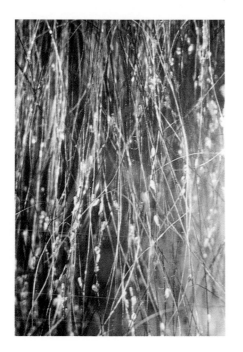

Figure 3.47 Lice infestation (head lice): numerous nits can be seen on these scalp hairs. Lice infestation usually presents in children with itching, and secondary infection over the nape of the neck. Head lice and nits (egg capsules) will be visible on careful examination. All scalps in the household or classroom should be checked and treated if necessary. Carbaryl lotion (0.5%), malathion lotion (0.5%), or phenothrin liquid (0.5%) are recommended; shampooing and combing after single applications of any of these pediculicides are an important part of the treatment. Simply shampooing and combing every 3 days should then be carried out.

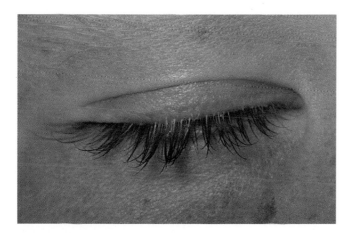

Figure 3.48 Lice infestation (pubic lice): nits are present on the eyelashes in this 5½-year-old girl. The parents attended clinic with her and the father said that he had had pubic lice and the daughter had slept in his bed when the mother was ill in hospital for a few days. There was no evidence of sexual abuse but there was obviously close physical contact between father and child. White soft paraffin was applied to the lashes as therapy.

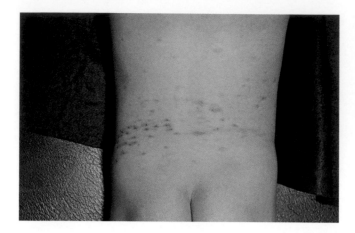

Figure 3.49 Insect bites: flea bites visible over left hip. Bites from human, bird, cat, or dog fleas, appear in the young as groups, often linear, or erythematous macular lesions, each with a central punctum. They are often noticed in the morning on awakening.

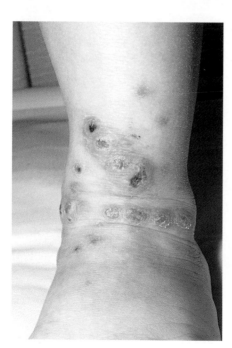

Figure 3.50 Insect bites: a boy of 19 months old with secondarily infected insect bites of florid eroded appearance over the lower leg, which were acquired on a holiday abroad in a warm climate.

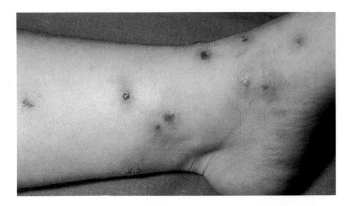

Figure 3.51 Papular urticaria: a typical site over the leg showing vesicles (some secondarily infected). Papular urticaria is more common than actual insect bites in children. It is rare in the first year of life. It represents a hypersensitivity reaction to a bite from a flea, bed bug, mosquito, or dog louse. Irritation, vesicles, papules, and weals appear over the buttocks and limbs, but distribution may be wider in chronic papular urticaria, and secondary infection of lesions is common. Usually, only one child in a family is affected and the eruption tends to reappear for a few years in the summer. Time is well spent explaining the condition to parents. An oral antihistamine and topical hydrocortisone combined with antiseptic or antibiotic are useful in management.

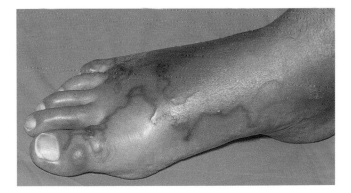

Figure 3.52 Creeping eruption: young adult with a striking eruption acquired in Barbados. This is a tortuous linear eruption usually caused by larvae of the dog or cat hookworm. Infections are most common in warm, humid and sandy coastal areas of tropical and subtropical regions. The larvae penetrate human skin that has been in contact with contaminated sandy areas and they remain in the skin producing a characteristic serpentine track. The condition is self-limiting but topical thiabendazole (10–15% for a few days) can be used in treatment and oral therapy, such as a single dose of albendazole, may be required.

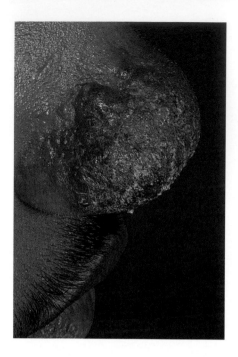

Figure 3.53 Cutaneous leishmaniasis: a Yemenite boy of 14 years old with an unsightly swollen erythematous nose. He responded to intravenous sodium stibogluconate. This is an infective granuloma of skin and subcutaneous tissues. The infestation is common among inhabitants of the Mediterranean, Middle East, India and South America and those who travel to these areas. The infection is caused by sandflies and the parasite involved is a protozoon. Incubation period following the bite varies from weeks to months. Lesions may be single or multiple and have a tendency to heal with scarring within a year. Treatment for extensive or unsightly lesions is with a systemic antimony compound as in this boy.

FURTHER READING

Burns DA. Infestations in schoolchildren. *Prescribers' Journal* 1998; **38**: 80–6.

Farrell AM. Staphylococcal scalded-skin syndrome. *Lancet* 1999; **354**: 880–81.

Hobbs CJ, Wynne J. How to manage warts. *Arch Dis Child* 1999: **81**; 460.

Ladhani S, Evans RW. Staphylococcal scalded skin syndrome. *Arch Dis Child* 1998; **78**: 85–8.

Pollard AJ, Faust SN, Levin M. Meningitis and meningococcal septicaemia *J Roy Coll Phys Lond* 1998; **32**: 319–28.

Verbov J. How to manage warts. *Arch Dis Child* 1999; **80**: 97–9.

4

Erythemato-squamous Disorders and Napkin-area Eruptions

CONTENTS

INTRODUCTION

Psoriasis (Figures 4.1–4.12, 4.33) is a common inherited condition but onset before the age of 5 years is unusual and before the age of 2 is rare: follow-up of patients with such early onset psoriasis indicates that lesions tend to be persistent and remissions are few and far between. It is a source of much discomfort and embarrassment. Typical lesions are discrete erythematous patches with overlying silvery scales.

Compliance with treatment must always be emphasized to the child's parents, to whom the condition should also be explained. In my experience, before puberty it is twice as common in girls with an equal sex incidence later; indicating that onset tends to be earlier in females. Coal tar-containing preparations (often with salicylic acid), calcipotriol (a vitamin D derivative) and dithranol (anthralin) preparations used carefully and initially in low concentration are useful topical applications in psoriasis. In my experience psoriatic arthropathy is uncommon in children.

Pityriasis rosea (Figures 4.13–4.14) will usually be managed by the Family Practitioner, but can sometimes go unrecognized or be confused with psoriasis. A clue to the diagnosis of this self-limiting condition in older children is often the fact that the rash has disappeared by the time the child attends for an early appointment.

Erythemato-squamous disorders

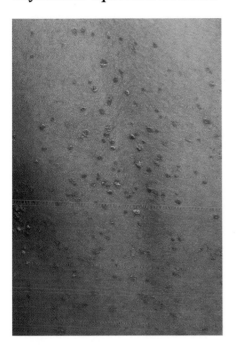

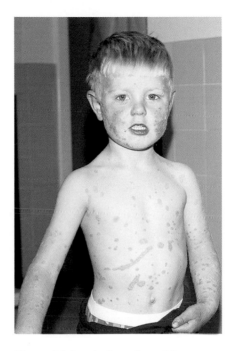

Figure 4.1 Psoriasis: a 5½-year-old boy with *guttate* psoriasis over the back. This is a common form of psoriasis in children. Guttate lesions often follow a streptococcal tonsillitis or other infection. The guttate eruption usually persists for only 3–4 months and then spontaneously resolves; the degree of itching is variable. However, it is common for psoriasis of some type to recur within the following 3–5 years or sooner. Mild short-lasting guttate psoriasis can often be managed with emollients alone.

Figure 4.2 Psoriasis: a boy of 5-years-old showing both guttate (drop-like) and larger (*plaque*) lesions and the *Köbner* phenomenon. In the Köbner phenomenon lesions appear along the site of injury, such as a scratch, and it is seen characteristically in active psoriasis (and in some other conditions such as molluscum contagiosum (see Figure 3.19), warts and lichen planus).

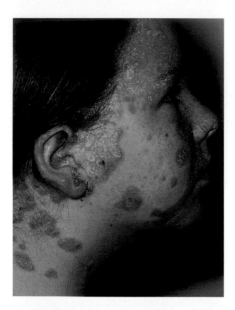

Figure 4.3 Psoriasis: plaque psoriasis over the face and neck with some spread into the external ear in a 14-year-old girl who had extensive psoriasis.

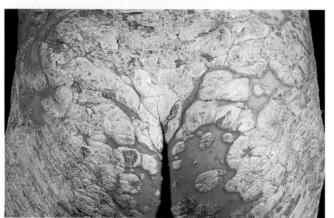

Figure 4.4 Psoriasis: severe buttock involvement in a boy with untreated lesions.

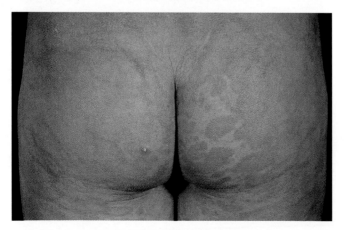

Figure 4.5 Psoriasis: the same boy as shown in Figure 4.4 following 18 days of treatment with topical dithranol in Lassar's paste only.

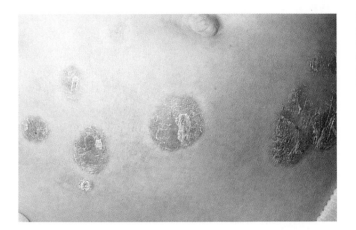

Figure 4.6 Psoriasis: plaques are visible over the trunk, some showing a surrounding halo – the ring of Woronoff.

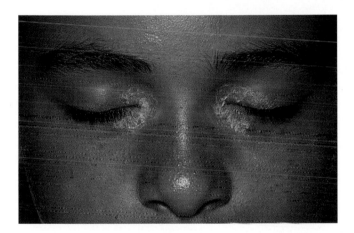

Figure 4.7 Psoriasis: typical psoriasis at an unusual site. His skin was clear elsewhere.

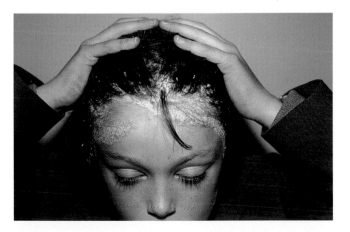

Figure 4.8 Psoriasis: severe scalp involvement in an 11-year-old boy. Patchy thick scaling areas are typical of scalp psoriasis and when scales are removed some hair may be lost but almost always re-grows.

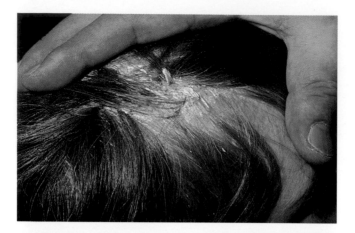

Figure 4.9 Psoriasis: a child with *pityriasis amiantacea*, a condition in which scalp patches occur showing white asbestos-like scales which cling firmly to hair shafts as they emerge from the scalp and extend some distance along them. Such hair will come away if gently pulled. In children, pityriasis amiantacea is often part of psoriasis but it may occur as a separate entity.

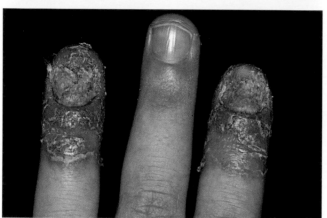

Figure 4.10 Psoriasis: a 7½-year-old girl with *pustular* psoriasis involving the skin and nails of two fingers only. Pustular psoriasis usually affects the palms and soles, and is relatively rare in children.

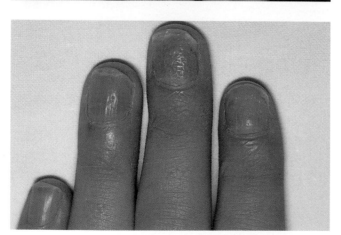

Figure 4.11 Psoriasis: the same girl shown in Figure 4.10 20 months later. Nail changes are seen particularly in chronic psoriasis and are uncommon in children. However, onycholysis (separation of the free end of the nail plate from the nail bed) and pitting may occur as seen here. Note that the middle finger which was unaffected by pustular psoriasis shows the most marked pitting. Nail changes in psoriasis occasionally occur *without* skin involvement.

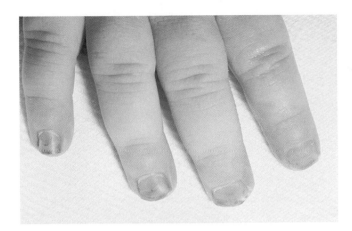

Figure 4.12
Psoriasis:
onycholysis in a 14-month-old infant who had plaque psoriasis elsewhere.

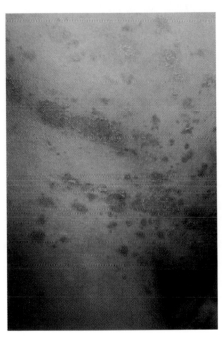

Figure 4.13 Pityriasis rosea: a boy of 5 years old with discrete superficial scaling lesions, some showing typical central scaling. This condition is a presumed virus infection, of 4–6 weeks duration, most commonly affecting older children and young adults. The first lesion is often larger and termed the *herald patch* and precedes others by a few days; the rash is typically irritant after a bath. Superficial scaly patches with increased scaling from the centre appear, particularly over the trunk, sometimes noticeably in the line of the ribs over the posterior rib cage. Occasionally in acute cases, papular, vesicular or purpuric lesions can occur. Maximum incidence is in the months November to February.

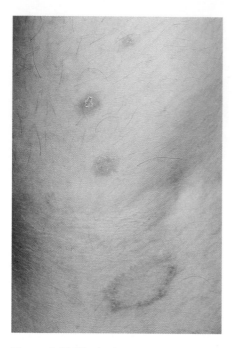

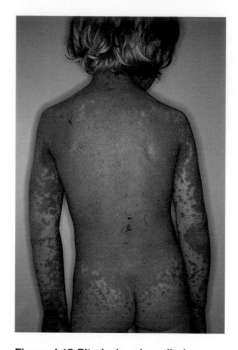

Figure 4.14 Pityriasis rosea: a close-up to show scaling lesions around the popliteal fossa.

Figure 4.15 Pityriasis rubra pilaris: a boy 4½ years old with widespread involvement. He had reddened skin but some unaffected areas over upper limbs are visible. This is a rare condition of unknown cause. It may present as a widespread psoriasiform eruption, in which small areas of normal-appearing skin are visible, or with marked skin thickening over the palms and soles showing orange–red discoloration. Patches over the knees will show follicular papules with hyperkeratotic plugs giving a rough feel. Frequently spontaneous remission occurs after months or even years.

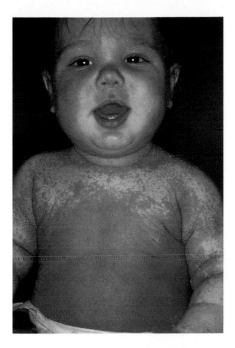

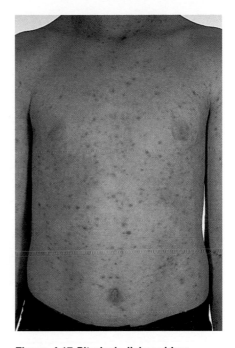

Figure 4.16 Pityriasis rubra pilaris: an infant with red skin but unaffected areas over the upper chest and upper arms are visible.

Figure 4.17 Pityriasis lichenoides: showing widespread haemorrhagic-looking papular eruption over the trunk. This is an uncommon self-limiting vasculitis. The basic lesion is a reddish-brown papule and lesions are most marked over the trunk and limbs. Lesions may be haemorrhagic, necrotic or show a removable central scale. There is no systemic upset and itching is minimal. It may persist for months or longer but tends to be of shorter duration in children than in adults. Exposure to UVB light or sunshine may hasten resolution.

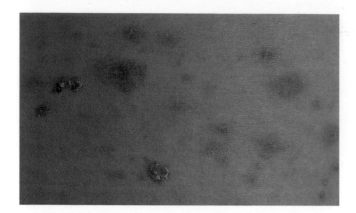

Figure 4.18 Pityriasis lichenoides: a close-up of lesions in an 11-year-old.

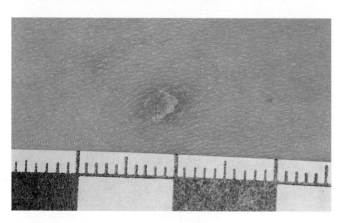

Figure 4.19 Pityriasis lichenoides: lesions showing typical mica (crumb-like) scale.

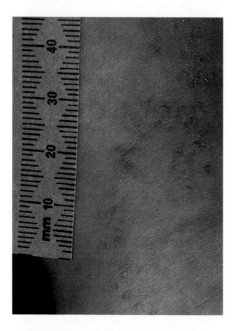

Figure 4.20 Lichen planus: a 20-month-old child with somewhat linear violaceous eruption over the left shin and medial ankle only. This condition of unknown cause is uncommon in children. Flat-topped violaceous papules appear, typically over front of wrist and trunk. There may be mouth and nail involvement. The picture illustrates a linear form.

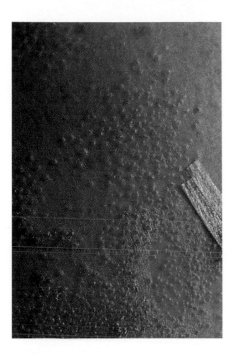

Figure 4.21 Lichen nitidus: an 8-year-old boy showing grouped small flat-topped papules over the trunk. Eruption resolved spontaneously. This is an uncommon self-limiting disorder seen particularly in children and can be considered a variant of lichen planus. It shows histological features identical to lichen planus yet more focal in nature. Small non-irritant papules occur in groups over the trunk.

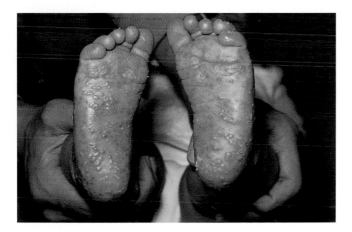

Figure 4.22 Acropustulosis of infancy: pustules over the sole in a 5-month-old boy. His mother was of West Indian origin. This condition seems to be more common in black infants. It occurs between the ages of 2–10 months. Crops of pruritic erythematous papules appear over palms and soles particularly, becoming vesico-papular, and they subside over a week or so only to recur a few weeks later. Scabies has to be excluded in the differential diagnosis but acropustulosis does seem to be a definite entity. Antihistamines help to reduce severe itching and the condition tends to resolve in the first 2–3 years of life.

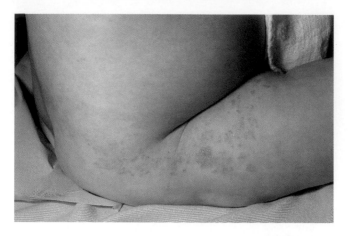

Figure 4.23 Asymmetric periflexural exanthem: superficial erythemato-squamous eruption is visible over thigh and slightly over adjacent trunk in an 11-month-old infant. This occurs in infancy, is more common in girls and usually resolves within a month. It tends to begin near the axilla and remains unilateral. *Lichen striatus* mentioned in Chapter 2 tends to affect older children, persists longer and linear bands generally predominate.

Napkin area eruptions

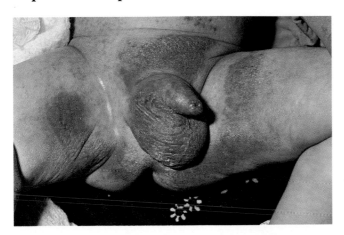

Figure 4.24 Napkin (diaper) dermatitis: W-shaped irritant dermatitis sparing groins. This is an irritant frictional contact dermatitis which is the most common eruption in the napkin area but has become less common, presumably due to modern rapidly-absorbent disposable nappies which result in less prolonged urine contact with the skin. Initially, the eruption is most prominent at sites of napkin contact and thus erythema and more severe inflammation will affect convexities. It usually appears after the first month of life probably because repeated skin insult is required before an eruption becomes obvious. It may occur alone or with other napkin area eruptions. Urea-splitting organisms in faeces or infected urine increase the alkalinity and likelihood of dermatitis. Soiled napkins left on for prolonged periods, or diarrhoea, encourage appearance of the dermatitis. The best treatment of napkin dermatitis is by exposure, if practical, but emollients or mildly-potent steroid applications are important too.

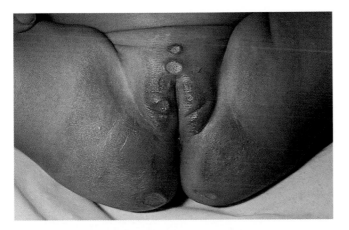

Figure 4.25 Napkin dermatitis: a more severe erosive type. This infant had an ammoniacal dermatitis: this old term should be correctly applied only to some eroded forms.

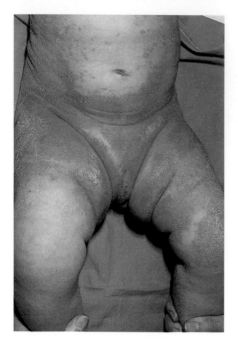

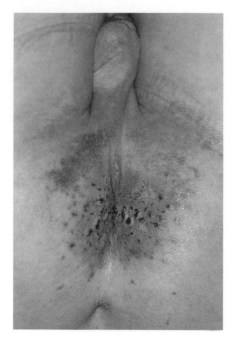

Figure 4.26 Napkin dermatitis: spreading scald appearance over the napkin area.

Figure 4.27 Napkin dermatitis: this 2-year-old boy had an herpetiform rather warty-looking irritant eruption mainly in the perianal region which followed surgery for Hirschsprung's disease. It was persistent but gradually improved. It is important to distinguish such an eruption from herpes simplex and viral warts.

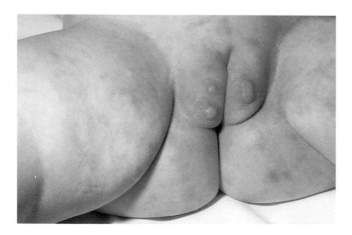

Figure 4.28 Infantile gluteal granuloma: a 10-month-old infant with typical soft nodules involving the vulva. There is a background of irritant dermatitis. This condition describes erythematous nodules appearing on a background of irritant dermatitis. The appearance sometimes may be related to abuse of topical steroids. Nodules spontaneously resolve but may take months to do so.

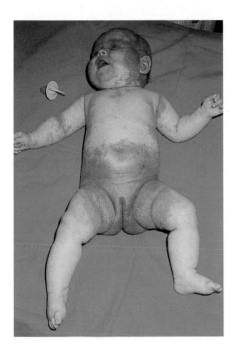

Figure 4.29 Infantile seborrhoeic dermatitis: classical involvement of the napkin area, axillae and scalp. This is non-irritant and typically occurs within the first three or four months of life clearing within weeks of onset. The napkin area, and particularly groins, or the scalp, are the common sites of onset but axillae, neck, and post-auricular regions are also usually affected. Erythema, maceration, and scaling involve the skin folds and the adjacent areas, but eruption becomes more widespread over the trunk and face. Yellowish, greasy scalp scaling (cradle cap) may be the only manifestation in some infants, yet occasionally in others a generalized erythroderma can occur. Local candidal and bacterial infections may complicate infantile seborrhoeic dermatitis and oral candidosis may also be present. There may be an increased incidence of atopy appearing later in these children. The relationship, if any, between this condition and seborrhoeic dermatitis in adolescents or adults (see Chapter 2) is unclear.

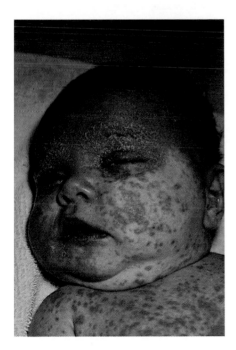

Figure 4.30 Infantile seborrhoeic dermatitis: severe facial and scalp involvement in a 1-month-old baby. Application of topical preparations containing a combination of hydrocortisone and either nystatin or an imidazole cream are useful. Scalp scaling can be treated with a cream containing sulphur (1%), salicylic acid (1%) in aqueous cream BP for a week or so.

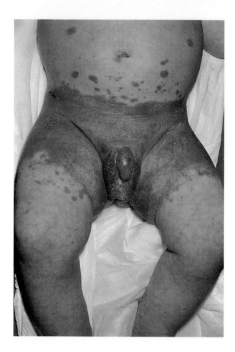

Figure 4.31 Napkin psoriasis: note the well-defined napkin area eruption with psoriasiform spread over the trunk. This is a form of *infantile seborrhoeic dermatitis* but it has been suggested that such children are more likely to develop psoriasis later.

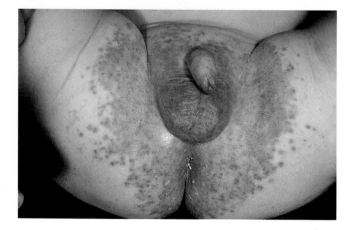

Figure 4.32 Candidosis: typical satellite pustules are visible as well as the main eruption. This presents as a moist erythema often with satellite pustules, over the buttocks and perianal region. Oral antibiotics predispose to the condition which can be treated with topical nystatin or an imidazole cream and treatment for oral candidosis, if necessary, also.

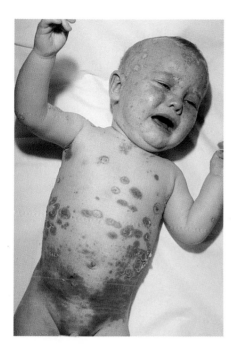

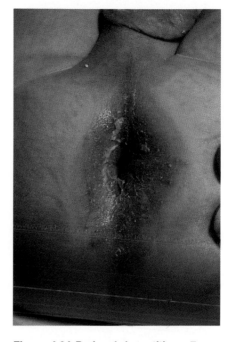

Figure 4.33 Psoriasis: an 8-month-old infant with true psoriasis which began at the age of 7 weeks. Note the typical psoriatic scaling over trunk and particularly forehead.

Figure 4.34 Perianal dermatitis: a 7-month-old boy with streptococcal skin sepsis elsewhere. Transient localized perianal dermatitis is common after diarrhoea but may form part of an irritant dermatitis or infantile seborrhoeic dermatitis. Streptococcal infection (including beta-haemolytic streptococci) is not an uncommon finding in perianal dermatitis and should be treated.

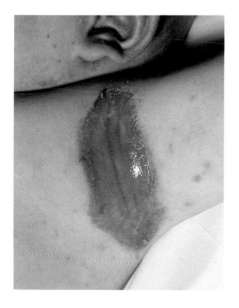

Figure 4.35 Intertrigo: this just involved the axillae in this overweight child. Intertrigo is a moist erythematous eruption where there is friction between opposed surfaces. Groins, neck and axillae are common sites. Affected infants are often overweight and unlike infantile seborrhoeic dermatitis the eruption is localized to the frictional site.

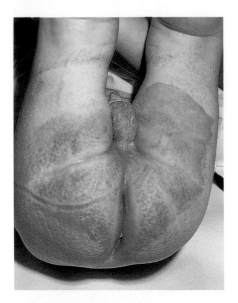

Figure 4.36 Drug eruption: note the well-defined distribution of the eruption where excreted drug has been spread by a soiled nappy. This was due to a danthron-containing stimulant laxative and skin staining is a drug side-effect.

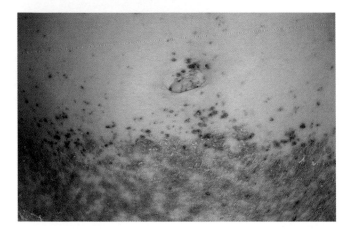

Figure 4.37 Langerhans cell histiocytosis: a close-up of a purpuric papular eruption involving the lower trunk. This condition has been mentioned in Chapter 1. It usually presents with an infantile seborrhoeic dermatitis-like picture but on closer inspection the reddish-brown or purpuric papules that are present differentiate it from a dermatitis.

FURTHER READING

Burden AD. Management of psoriasis in childhood. *Clin Exp Dermatol* 1999; **24**: 341–45.

Mancini AJ, Frieden IJ, Paller AS. Infantile acropustulosis revisited: history of scabies and response to topical corticosteroids. *Pediatr Dermatol* 1998; **15**: 337–41.

Mendelsohn SS, Verbov JL. Asymmetric periflexural exanthem of childhood. *Clin Exp Dermatol* 1994; **19**: 421.

Rodriguez-Poblador J, González-Castro U, Herranz-Martinez S, Luelmo-Aguilar J. Jacquet erosive diaper dermatitis after surgery for Hirschsprung disease. *Pediatr Dermatol* 1998; **15**: 46–7.

Verbov J. Psoriasis in childhood. *Arch Dis Child* 1992; **67**: 75–6.

5

Hair and Nails

CONTENTS

INTRODUCTION

Scalp hair loss will be an understandable cause for concern to parents and older children. There are very many causes of scalp hair loss and sometimes more than one cause is present. A common condition such as nail biting will rarely be referred for a consultant opinion and similarly chronic paronychia due to finger sucking can be managed in the community.

Hair loss

Figure 5.1 Alopecia areata: extensive hair loss over posterior scalp in an 8-year-old. Alopecia areata is a common cause of hair loss in children and the commonest type of hair fall seen in my clinics. It is a cause of much distress to both child and family and time spent explaining the condition to parents is well-spent. Hairless smooth areas of skin, usually over the scalp, are visible; remnants of broken-off hairs, visible as 'exclamation marks', may be seen at the edge of active patches. Early patches may show an irregular outline. Prognosis is good when there are few patches of hair loss, with a likely regrowth in 6–12 months, and both parents and child should be told this, but the more extensive the loss the more guarded should be the prognosis; occipital hair regrows more slowly. When associated with atopy the prognosis tends to be poor. The condition is sometimes recurrent.

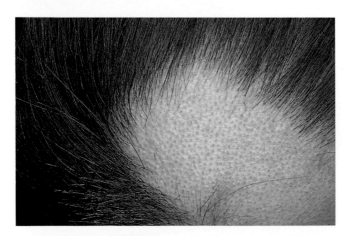

Figure 5.2 Alopecia areata: a close-up of an area of alopecia, showing 'exclamation mark' hairs between 9 and 2 o'clock.

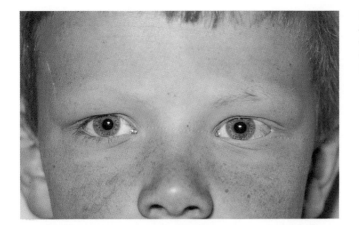

Figure 5.3 Alopecia areata: the left eyelashes and right eyebrow hair were lost in this 8-year-old boy.

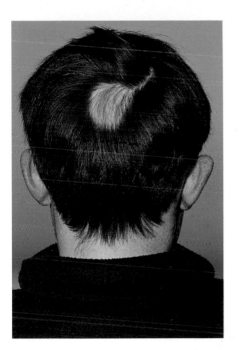

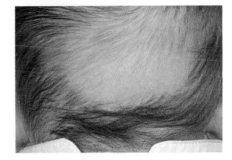

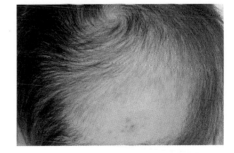

Figure 5.4 Alopecia areata: re-growing lighter coloured hair in an area of alopecia areata. New hair is often lighter, showing normal pigmentation in time.

Figure 5.5 Physiological: occipital hair loss in 7-month-old twin brothers. Such occipital hair loss is usual in infants and is temporary. It is due to a combination of movement, pressure, and alteration in hair cycle (delayed telogen).

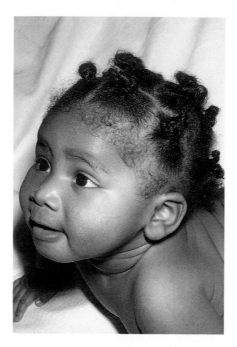

Figure 5.6 Trauma (unintentional hair loss): a 7-month-old Jamaican girl with traction alopecia. Traumatic hair loss may be unintentional or intentional and may be self-inflicted or caused by another person or object. Pony tails, various ethnic hair styles, some fashionable hair styles, tight rollers and hot combs may cause patchy alopecia unintentionally.

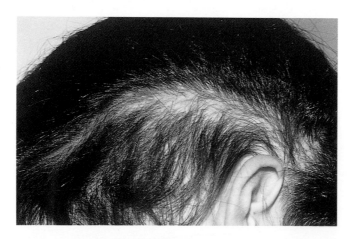

Figure 5.7 Trauma (unintentional hair loss): in a 13-year-old girl with traction alopecia over the right side of her scalp.

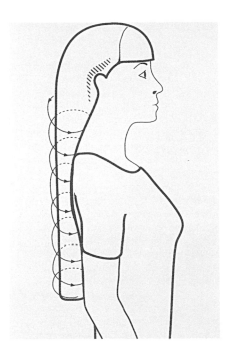

Figure 5.8 Trauma (unintentional hair loss): the same girl as shown in Figure 5.7 with a diagram illustrating how the hair-twisting and pulling of her long pony tail to the left side resulted in pulling of the hair above her right ear and subsequent hair loss. Her hair re-grew rapidly after the cause was explained to her.

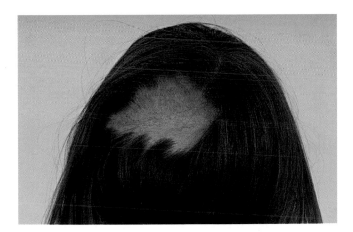

Figure 5.9 Trauma (unintentional hair loss): a 4-year-old girl whose hair got caught up in a food mixer when she sat on a table with her back to the machine when it was turned on, with her hair hanging down. The torn-off patch re-grew normally.

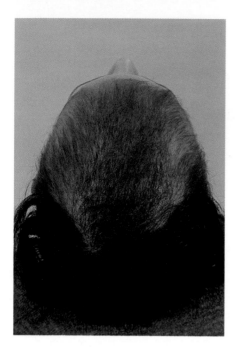

Figure 5.10 Trauma (intentional hair loss): bizarre, widespread *trichotillomania* in a 9-year-old girl with hair of normal appearance persisting at the sides and posterior scalp. All her traumatized hair re-grew within a year. *Trichotillomania* is the term sometimes used to describe a self-inflicted form of traumatic alopecia. Children may cause breakage of hairs by twisting groups of hairs, or they can pull out, or rarely cut or shave their own hair intentionally. Usually of no lasting consequence, it can be important if persistent and extensive; chronic social deprivation is not an uncommon trigger. It may also be a manifestation of anxiety, obsession–compulsion or depression. Differentiation from alopecia areata is usually based on the irregular outline of the alopecia in self-inflicted hair loss, its bizarre appearance and the presence of short stub-like hairs. The approach to the child with suspected intentional, self-inflicted hair loss should be very circumspect: such children should not be accused of pulling out the hair (in any case they will often deny this). Rapport with the child and parent must be gained over a few consultations. It is interesting that trichotillomania *may follow* alopecia areata: perhaps the attention the child with alopecia areata receives may make the occasional individual pull out his/her hair later to gain attention.

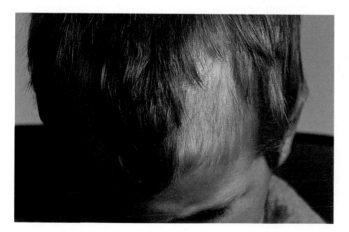

Figure 5.11 Trauma (intentional hair loss): self-inflicted hair loss over the anterior scalp. This 5½-year-old boy was unhappy in school and admitted that he was pulling out his hair. His situation was resolved and the hair re-grew but he then began to bite his nails. Such hair loss is more common in boys at this age, but it is more common in females in older individuals.

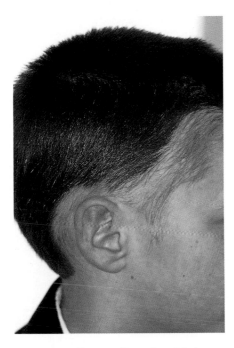

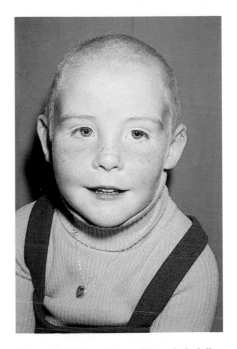

Figure 5.12 Trauma (intentional hair loss): self-inflicted hair loss over the sides of the scalp. This boy told me that he pulled his hair out when he was bored at school.

Figure 5.13 Hereditary diffuse hair fall: a young girl with sparse scalp hairs as an isolated finding. Such hair loss may occur by itself, sometimes as an autosomal dominant trait, and is usually permanent. However, sparse scalp hair is more commonly just one sign in ectodermal dysplasias, acrodermatitis enteropathica and other conditions.

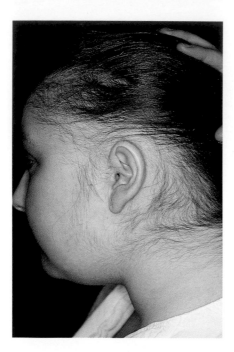

Figure 5.14 Systemic disease: this adolescent girl presented with scalp hair loss, obesity and increasing lethargy; she had *hypothyroidism* which responded rapidly to therapy.

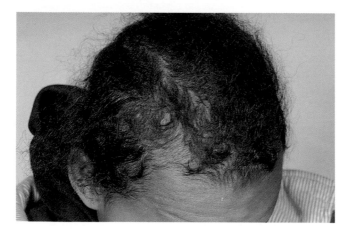

Figure 5.15 Systemic disease: this girl with scalp hair loss was found to have *diabetes mellitus*.

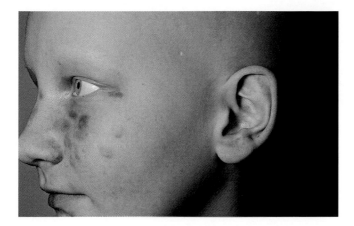

Figure 5.16 Systemic disease therapy: this girl of 14 years old developed complete hair fall due to chemotherapy prescribed for rhabdomyosarcoma. Such toxic hair fall is termed *anagen effluvium* and usually regrows after chemotherapy.

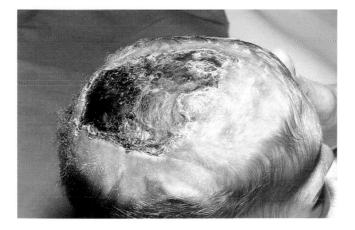

Figure 5.17 Scarring alopecia: a male infant with an extensive congenital scalp skin defect (*aplasia cutis*). He also had cardiac defects which required surgical correction. Scarring alopecia is the end result of many processes, often inflammatory, resulting in irreversible scarring of the affected area. Local infections, trauma and various skin conditions may produce scarring. *Aplasia cutis* (Figures 5.17 and 5.18) is a rare congenital developmental abnormality resulting in scarring. In some cases it is genetically determined, and most commonly affects the scalp: a crust or ulcer present at birth heals, leaving a scar. The depth of such scalp tissue loss should be assessed because deeper tissue including bone can, rarely, also be absent. Thus, aplasia cutis is one of the many causes of scarring alopecia. Note that congenital absence of skin may also be due to trauma.

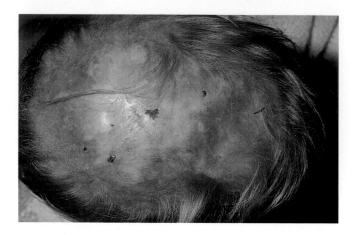

Figure 5.18 Scarring alopecia: the same boy as shown in Figure 5.17 with aplasia cutis at the age of 3 years old showing healed atrophic scar over scalp. He protected his scalp from trauma in infancy with a helmet and later as the defect area contracted a rubber skull cap. He later had plastic surgery to excise much of the scar and bring hair bearing scalp skin together to close the area with an expanding technique.

Hair shaft deformities

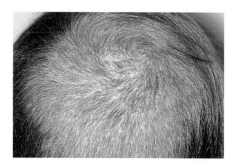

Figure 5.19 Monilethrix: a child of 14 years old with scalp hair thinning and showing the typical beaded hairs. Monilethrix is an autosomal dominant permanent condition affecting scalp hairs and producing partial alopecia. Individual hairs show beading with the elliptical nodes 0.7–1.0 mm apart separated by narrow internodes at which the medulla is missing. The internodes break transversely so that hair fails to grow to any appreciable length.

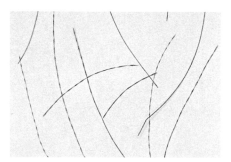

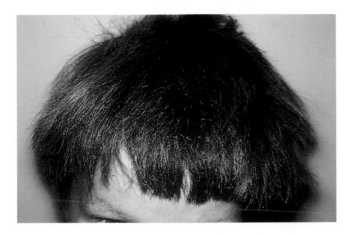

Figure 5.20 Pili torti (twisting of hair): the flickering effect on hairs with reflected light at the site of the twists is seen over the anterior scalp. Pili torti indicates multiple 180° twists, each no more than a fraction of a millimetre long, affecting the scalp hair particularly. It can occur alone as an isolated autosomal dominant condition or in other inherited syndromes. When light is shone on twisted hair at varying angles, a flecking or spangling effect is seen.

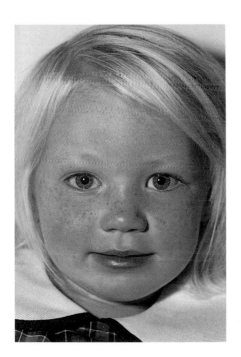

Figure 5.21 Loose anagen: a child with blonde hair whose hair could be painlessly plucked and who presented with diffuse hair loss. This condition is seen mainly in young girls, often with blonde hair. Spontaneous resolution is common.

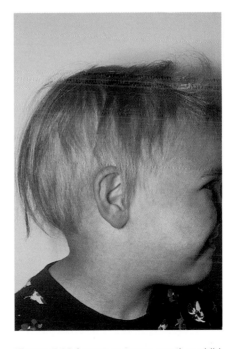

Figure 5.22 Loose anagen: another child with more marked hair loss which re-grew spontaneously.

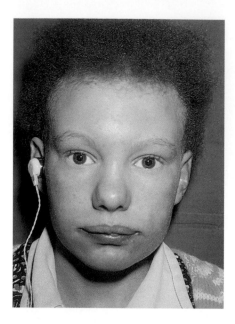

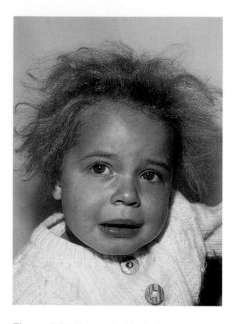

Figure 5.23 Woolly hair: this 13-year-old girl has the wiry, woolly scalp hair of the woolly hair syndrome. In addition she had congenital perceptive deafness and ichthyosis vulgaris. Woolly hair syndrome may occur as a localized hair naevus, or as a congenital inherited condition in caucasians affecting the whole scalp and giving the appearance of afro-caribbean hair. It is usually autosomal dominant but may be recessive. Hairs tend to break easily with minor trauma.

Figure 5.24 Uncombable hair syndrome: since birth this 2½-year-old girl had unruly hair which slowly improved. This syndrome is usually first noticed at around the age of 3 years. The scalp hair is disorderly and remains so despite brushing and combing. Hair shafts on microscopy show a longitudinal depression and may be triangular. Spontaneous improvement is usual.

Nails

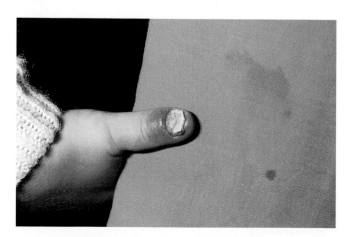

Figure 5.25 Chronic paronychia: inflamed nail folds with dystrophic nail in a thumb-sucker. This is seen most commonly in digit suckers or biters. A mixed flora of bacteria and Candida is often found. The skin is usually erythematous, slightly swollen and shiny with a nail deformity present.

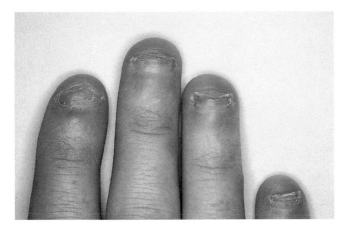

Figure 5.26 Nail biting: showing bitten finger nails. Nail biting is a common habit. Children should be warned that permanent damage to the nail will occur if the nail matrix (situated under the posterior nail fold and from which the nail derives) is damaged.

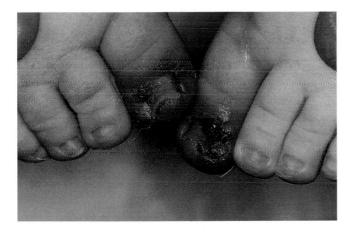

Figure 5.27 Ingrowing toe-nail: a 7-month-old infant with ingrowing big toe-nails, particularly laterally. Ingrowing toe-nail is not uncommon in childhood. In infants a combination of walking and pressure from ill-fitting footwear may induce pain, bacterial paronychia and overgrowth of granulation tissue around the soft pliable nail plate. In addition, incorrect cutting of the toenails is an important factor. However, a primary but self-limiting factor in infants can be unduly prominent skin at the extreme tip of the big toe forming an anterior nail fold which encourages ingrowing and prevents the free end of the big toe-nail growing normally. Local antiseptic measures will be required and advice to parents regarding avoidance of toe pressure trauma.

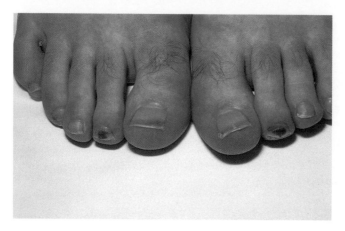

Figure 5.28 Haemorrhage: shown under the second toe-nails due to wearing a friend's smaller sized hockey boots. Haemorrhage under a nail may be due to obvious trauma but platform shoes, too tight shoes, or other fashionable-heeled shoes worn by older children not uncommonly cause haemorrhage under a nail (subungual haemorrhage) and the nail may separate later.

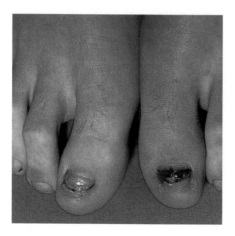

Figure 5.29 Haemorrhage: loss of big toe-nails due to platform shoe trauma – sliding down of the feet in the shoes.

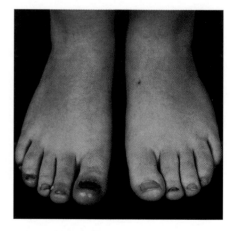

Figure 5.30 Pulled nails (onychotillomania): a girl of 14 years old who presented with loss of some toe-nails and haemorrhage around and under others. The condition resolved after a few years. She was unhappy at school with an art teacher who she felt had ostracized her for no reason. Self-inflicted toe-nail loss is rare and the patient never admitted that she traumatized the nails herself.

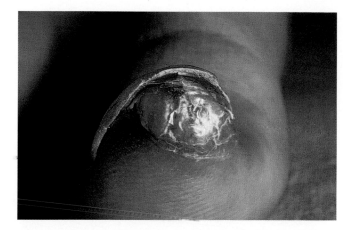

Figure 5.31 Subungual exostosis: note the nail lifted by the underlying swelling. This is a solitary bony outgrowth of the distal phalanx of a digit, particularly the big toe. Lesions may be due to trauma or appear spontaneously. A small flesh-coloured growth develops, and projects beyond the free edge of the nail, sometimes detaching the nail. It is often painful. Treatment is exclsion by an orthopaedic surgeon.

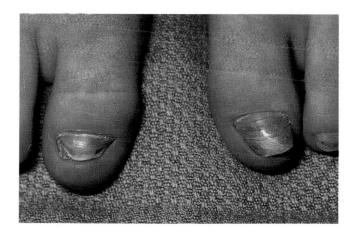

Figure 5.32 Malalignment of the big toe-nail: the left big toe-nail in this 8-year-old girl had been deviated laterally since the age of 1 year. Malalignment of the big toe-nail will encourage ingrowing of the nail. If lateral deviation of the nail plate is present and is marked, surgical correction with re-alignment of the whole nail apparatus may be indicated. However, spontaneous resolution of such malalignment does occur and in my experience patience is worthwhile.

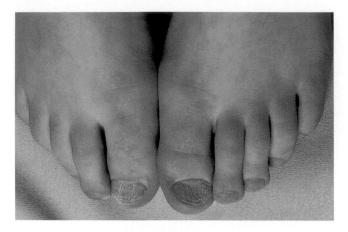

Figure 5.33 Twenty-nail dystrophy: opaque, longitudinally
ridged, deformed big toe nails. This is an acquired dystrophy
that begins in childhood. It is usually of unknown cause, but
may occur as part of alopecia areata or lichen planus. Excessive
longitudinal ridging, opacity, and either shininess or roughness
occur. It tends to be self-limiting and reversible although any nail
damage may persist.

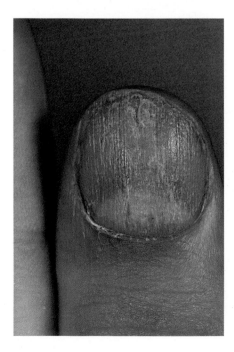

Figure 5.34 Twenty-nail dystrophy:
opaque, longitudinally ridged, thumb-nail
with transverse splitting of the free end
into layers, in a 10-year-old.

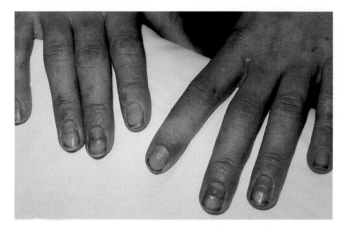

Figure 5.35 Beau's lines: this boy had had infectious mononucleosis a few months previously and that time is indicated by the position of transverse lines visible on some nails. Such lines are transverse depressions of the nails which appear as a reaction to any severe illness that temporarily interrupts nail formation. They become visible a few months after the onset of the illness. Since the lines originate under the proximal nail-fold, the date of the illness can be estimated by the distance of depression from the cuticle.

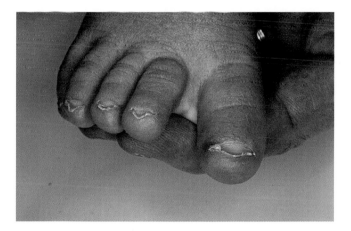

Figure 5.36 Koilonychia: an 11-month-old male infant showing spooned toe-nails. He had iron deficiency at times. Koilonychia is seen frequently as a normal finding in the first few months of life owing to the thin and soft nail plate. However, a dominant inherited form exists, and iron deficiency anaemia is a further cause of flat or spoon-shaped nails and sometimes no cause is found.

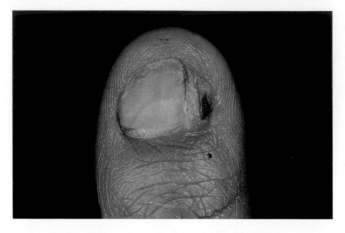

Figure 5.37 Nail-patella syndrome: Partial absence of right thumb-nail. This is an autosomal dominant condition in which small rudimentary patellae, elbow deformities, iliac spurs and abnormal nail formation occur; thumb-nails and index fingernails are particularly affected. Chronic glomerulonephritis occurs occasionally. Nails may be reduced in size or split longitudinally.

FURTHER READING

Ang P, Tay Y-K. What syndrome is this? (Uncombable hair syndrome). *Pediatr Dermatol* 1998; **15**: 475–76.

Baran R, Dawber RPR. The nail in childhood and old age. In: Baran R, Dawber RPR, eds. *Diseases of the Nails and their Management* 2nd edn. Oxford: Blackwell Science, 1994.

Baran R, Haneke L. Etiology and treatment of nail malalignment. *Dermatol Surg* 1998; **24**: 719–21.

Verbov J. Hair loss in children. *Arch Dis Child* 1993; **68**: 702–6.

6

Naevi, Other Developmental Abnormalities and Nodules

INTRODUCTION

Freckles are innocent and commonplace and are usually an incidental observation when a child attends with some other condition. Media publicity has made the general public more aware of the importance of pigmented naevi and of the dangers of over-exposure to the sun. Many children are referred when their moles have altered in size. However, this is usually because the mole has grown as the child has grown and is nothing to worry about. Halo naevus, in which a pale halo surrounds a mole, is a common benign phenomenon in childhood.

Pigmented naevi

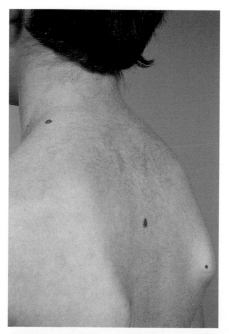

Figure 6.1 Melanocytic naevus: a child of 11 years old showing three naevi.
Melanocytic naevi composed of naevus cells, are divided into intradermal, junctional and compound types (depending on the location of the naevus cells). Only 1–3% of neonates have any such naevi at birth. These naevi, often referred to as *moles*, are very common and the majority appear in childhood and adolescence. Face, neck and back are the usual sites. It is rare in childhood for a mole to show malignant change.

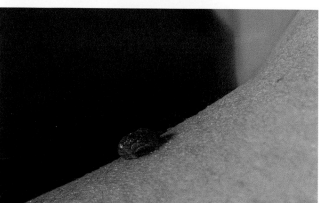

Figure 6.2
Melanocytic naevus: a close up of the same child as shown in Figure 6.1 showing a dome-shaped sessile intradermal naevus over the shoulder.

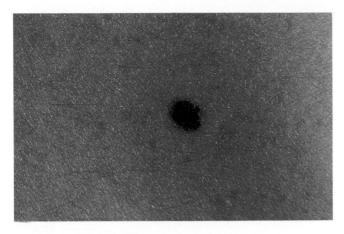

Figure 6.3 Melanocytic naevus: a close up of the same child as shown in Figures 6.1 and 6.2 showing a dark-brown, flat, hairless junctional naevus over the right scapula.

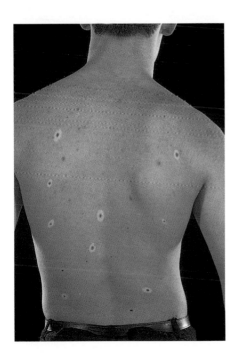

Figure 6.4 Halo naevus: a boy of 14 years old with multiple halo naevi. Halo naevus is a common single or multiple lesion which usually presents over the trunk with an area of depigmentation around a central, commonly compound melanocytic naevus. The cause of the depigmentation is unknown but there is an increased incidence of vitiligo (Chapter 11) in patients with such naevi. Both naevi and halo have a tendency to resolve spontaneously but this may take several years.

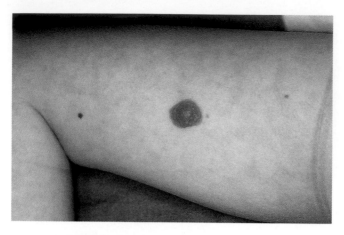

Figure 6.5 Spindle-cell naevus: a vascular-appearing orange–brown nodule over thigh. Spindle-cell naevus is a common lesion which presents as a smooth-surfaced dome-shaped nodule, often reddish brown, correlating with the vascularity of the benign tumour, but it may be black and can have a warty appearance. Cells are generally spindle-shaped and multinucleated giant cells and mitotic figures are also present. The spindle and giant cells are two features distinguishing the lesion from malignant melanoma. The lesion is usually excised to confirm the diagnosis.

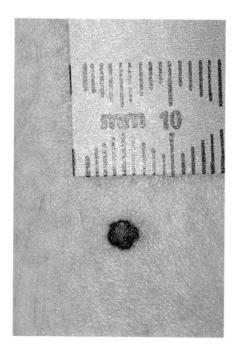

Figure 6.6 Spindle-cell naevus: a girl of 6 years old with lesion over her right thigh. This dark lesion shows an irregular edge and is somewhat warty. I considered excision essential just to confirm its benign nature.

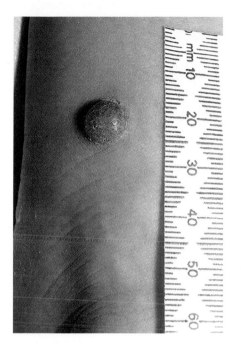

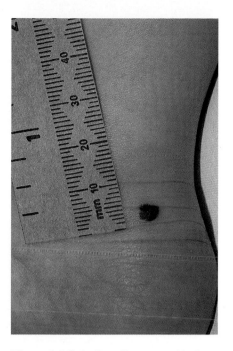

Figure 6.7 Spindle-cell naevus: a firm nodule over the dorsum foot.

Figure 6.8 Spindle-cell naevus: black, raised lesion just above the heel in a girl of almost 3 years. It had appeared at the age of 16 months. Excision confirmed the diagnosis.

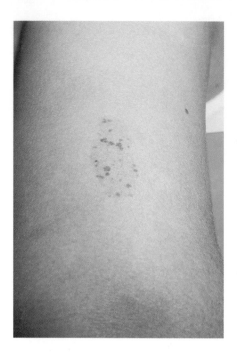

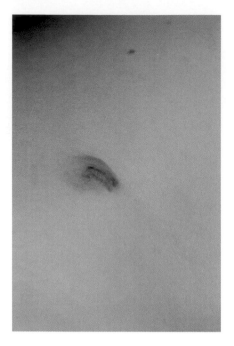

Figure 6.9 Naevus spilus: lesion over the upper arm showing dots of darker pigmentation both at the edge and within the background patch of macular brown pigmentation. This is a solitary brown macule dotted with small brownish–black areas of pigmentation. It may be 1cm or more in diameter.

Figure 6.10 Blue naevus: this shows the *common type* of blue naevus. This presents as an area of blue or blue–black dermal pigmentation, often slightly raised but smooth-surfaced, produced by aberrant localized collections of functioning melanocytes. Common sites are dorsa of the hands and feet, buttocks and face. Lesions may appear at any age. There are two types; the common type as shown here, and the cellular blue naevus (Figure 6.11) which tends to be larger than 1cm in diameter, and with a different histopathology.

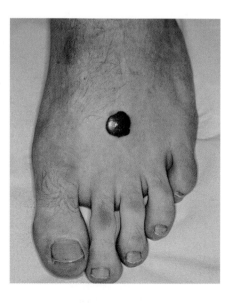

Figure 6.11 Blue naevus: this shows a *cellular* blue naevus. It was excised to exclude a malignant melanoma but was benign on histology.

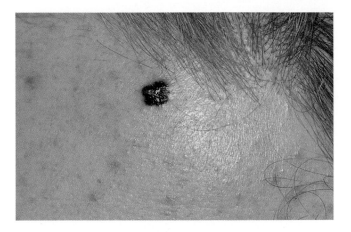

Figure 6.12 Malignant melanoma: a boy of 17 with an irregular-edged black nodule over forehead, present one year and enlarging. Change in shape, colour or size of a melanocytic naevus, other than with growth of the child, should alert the clinician to the possibility of malignant melanoma. Irregular-edged moles or moles with unusual features should mean referral to a specialist. Although very rare before puberty, such a diagnosis must not be forgotten in young adults. Children with *giant congenital pigmented naevi* (Chapter 1) are at an increased risk of developing melanoma.

Vascular naevi

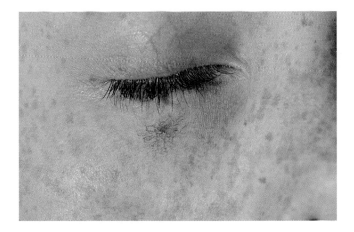

Figure 6.13 Spider naevus: a girl of 9 years old with spider naevus below right eye. A spider naevus consists of a central arteriole with radiating vessels. These are common lesions which occur on the upper half of the body. Lesions tend to persist. The central vessel can be destroyed, if necessary, by laser treatment, cautery, or diathermy in the older child. Occasionally, larger lesions may require excision.

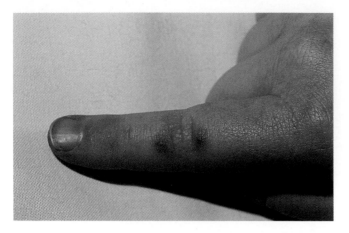

Figure 6.14 Spider naevus: two spider naevi over a finger in a girl of 7 years old.

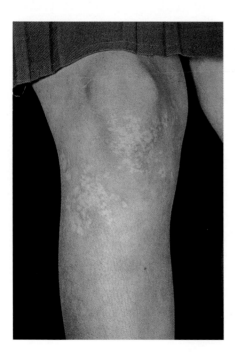

Figure 6.15 Naevus anaemicus: paler areas over and below the knee are visible. This lesion is a congenital skin anomaly, characterized by macular areas of skin pallor due to reduced blood flow. The lesion is a pharmacological one showing an increased vascular reactivity to circulating catecholamines. Such lesions are sometimes seen in association with *portwine stains* and they appear to be more frequent in *neurofibromatosis*.

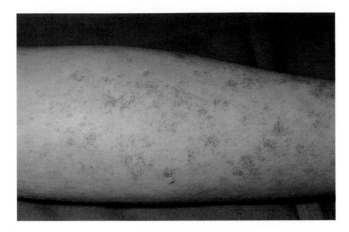

Figure 6.16 Angioma serpiginosum: a girl of 8 showing small vascular areas over limb. A rare disorder of upper dermal capillaries and venules which show localized dilatations. It occurs mainly in females and onset is usually in childhood. Lower limbs and buttocks are preferred sites. It begins as one or more red or purple puncta which extend over a period of months or years. Individual puncta may disappear but complete resolution is uncommon.

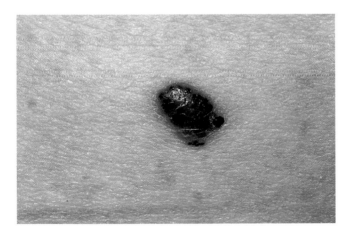

Figure 6.17 Lymphangioma circumscriptum: a 6-year-old boy with a vesicular-appearing black nodule over the abdomen with vesicles of frog spawn appearance at edge. This was surgically removed. Lymphangioma circumscriptum is the most common form of lymphangioma and presents at birth or in early childhood. It is characterized by groups of deep-seated thick-walled vesicles that resemble frog spawn. Frequently, there is an haemangiomatous element. Although 'circumscriptum', larger lesions particularly, may reveal a more widespread abnormality on investigation: this is very important if surgery is contemplated. Common sites are proximal limbs, chest wall and perineum.

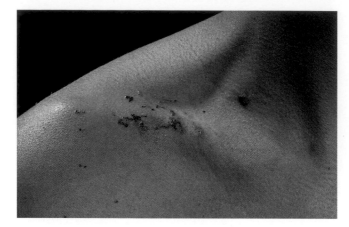

**Figure 6.18
Lymphangioma
circumscriptum:** a
boy of 14 years old
with vesicles, some of
which were
haemorrhagic, over
the right shoulder. The
lesion was of long
standing and
management
conservative.

Epidermal naevi

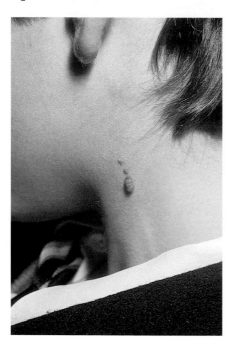

Figure 6.19 Verrucous naevus: localized
warty linear lesions over the neck. Epidermal
naevi of verrucous type may be localised or
widespread. Lesions present at birth or
appear in infancy or early childhood and
grow with the individual. They are skin-
coloured or brown, raised with a rough warty
surface. They vary in size and tend to be
linear when over limbs (see Chapter 1).
Histopathology shows hyperkeratosis,
papillomatosis, and acanthosis. If requiring
treatment excision is recommended because
cryotherapy, laser therapy, or cautery are
often followed by recurrence sooner or later.
One should not be tempted to advise
surgery at too early an age because the
naevus may continue to extend for some
years. Widespread lesions may form wavy
transverse bands on the trunk and
longitudinal, often spiral, streaks on the
limbs. Some of these show features of
epidermolytic hyperkeratosis on histology
and in some cases may be a manifestation
of that disorder (see Chapter 1). Extensive
unilateral verrucous naevi are sometimes
referred to as *naevus unius lateris*. Warty
naevi, usually of the widespread type, may
uncommonly be associated with
developmental defects in other systems and
such cases are referred to as the *epidermal
naevus syndrome.*

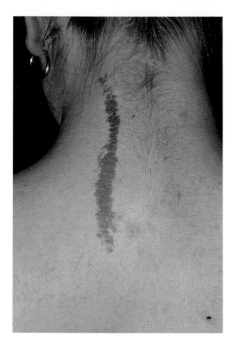

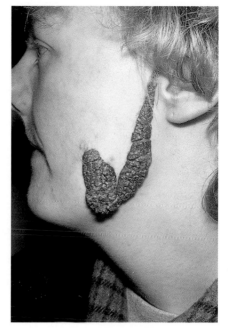

Figure 6.20 Verrucous naevus:
localized, linear, warty naevus over back
of the neck.

Figure 6.21 Verrucous naevus:
localized, well-defined lesion over face in
a 19-year-old. Although the lesion was
present for years, she waited until the age
of 19 years to have it dealt with by plastic
surgery, which produced an excellent
result.

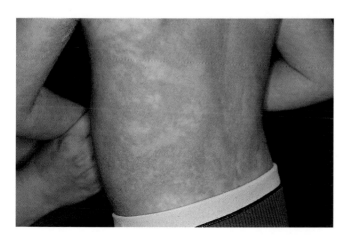

**Figure 6.22
Verrucous naevus:**
widespread naevus in
a 2½-year-old boy
which became more
verrucous and
widespread as he
grew.

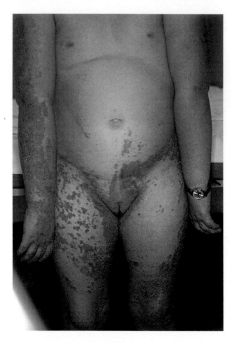

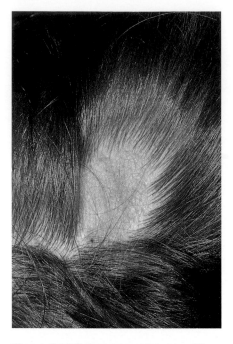

Figure 6.23 Inflamed linear epidermal naevus (eczematous epidermal naevus): a girl of 5 years old with an irritant psoriasiform eruption. This usually appears in infancy and is more common in females. It is pruritic and consists of scaly patches which look psoriasiform or eczematous and may appear warty. Most occur over lower limbs and buttocks and may be extensive. Histopathology reveals hyperkeratosis, parakeratosis, spongiosis and a dermal inflammatory infiltrate. Mild topical applications, often containing coal tar, can be applied.

Figure 6.24 Sebaceous naevus: a 3½-year-old girl with congenital, slightly raised, orange-looking, warty, hairless scalp patch. This lesion contains both epidermal and dermal elements. Most common over the scalp and usually single, it initially presents as smooth, slightly raised, hairless waxy plaques, yellowish-orange in colour and somewhat oval in shape. They thicken and become more elevated in late childhood and adolescence. Histologically there is an increase in the number of sebaceous glands which may also be enlarged and associated with hypertrophy and hyperkeratosis of the epidermis. Because benign or malignant change, particularly basal cell carcinoma, is not uncommon in these lesions, usually from the fourth decade, excision should be carried out as a precaution in early adult life.

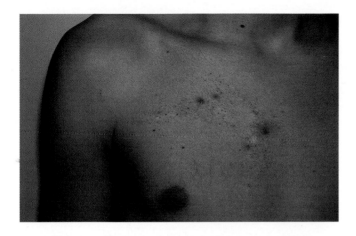

Figure 6.25 Comedone naevus: linear lesions over the upper chest showing blackheads and folliculitis. This usually appears by the age of 20 and may be present at birth. It consists of a group of dilated follicular orifices containing dark, horny plugs. The area affected may be 2 cm in diameter or more extensive. The face, neck, upper arm and chest are usual sites.

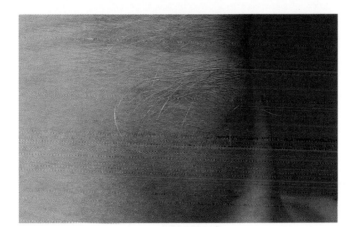

Figure 6.26 Naevoid hypertrichosis: white hair over the front of the neck in a girl of 5 years old. The condition was present since 7 months old and was treated by cutting at intervals. The presence of excess hair may occur as a developmental defect in the absence of any other abnormality.

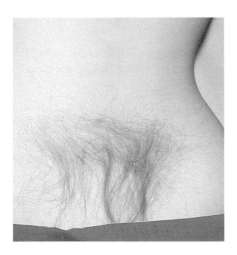

Figure 6.27 Faun-tail naevus: this child had no defect underlying the hair. An abnormal growth of hair (a faun-tail) or other skin lesion over the mid-line of the spine, usually in the sacral region, may indicate spina bifida. In view of the possible association of spinal cord abnormalities with spina bifida which may not produce symptoms until late childhood, the presence of any such skin lesions should lead to neurological assessment.

Other developmental abnormalities

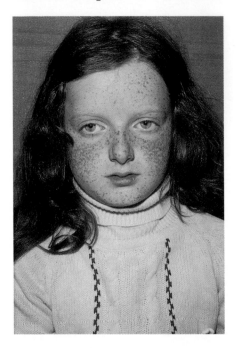

Figure 6.28 Freckles (ephelides): in a red-haired, fair-skinned child. These are light brown well-defined macules, usually less than 2 mm in diameter which usually appear in early childhood rather than infancy. There is no increase in melanocytes in the lesions. They occur especially on sun-exposed areas in fair or red-haired children and tend to fade somewhat in winter.

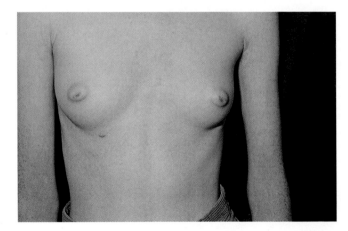

Figure 6.29 Supernumerary nipple: a 14-year-old girl with an extra nipple inferior to right breast. Such lesions develop along the course of the embryological milk lines which run from the anterior axillary folds to the inner thighs. They occur in both sexes. They can be confused with moles or viral warts if the diagnosis is not considered.

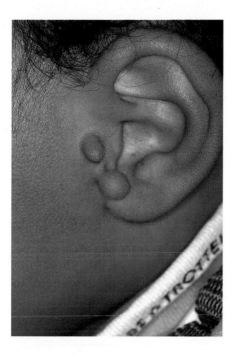

Figure 6.30 Auricular appendage: two such lesions anterior to the ear are visible in this 11-month-old infant. These common lesions appear anterior to the auricle and are usually unilateral, often on narrow pedicles. They usually consist of skin but may be broad-based and contain some cartilage.

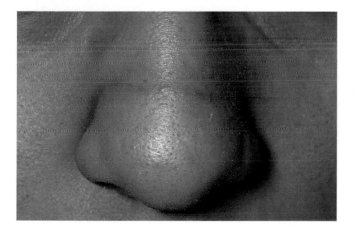

Figure 6.31 Nasal crease: transverse hyperpigmented area in an adolescent atopic boy. Such transverse nasal lesions which may be flat, grooved, or slightly raised are not uncommonly seen in childhood and may sometimes be associated with manipulation of the nose as a habit in those with allergic rhinitis. The site affected seems to be related to altered growth of nasal cartilages and this may make the individual more susceptible to developing the skin defect.

Nodules

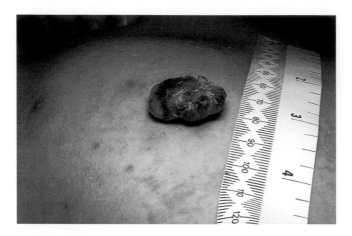

Figure 6.32 Granuloma telangiectaticum (pyogenic granuloma): easily bleeding vascular lesion over the chest, present at 6 months old. These vascular nodules develop rapidly often at the site of a recent trauma. They are usually dull red, fleshy and polypoid and may be pedunculated. They easily bleed with trauma. Treatment is curettage, followed by diathermy coagulation of the base but formal excision is sometimes required.

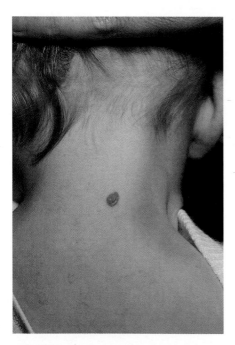

Figure 6.33 Juvenile xanthogranuloma: solitary, soft, yellowish–brown lesion over the back of the neck in 16-month-old boy. This is a self-limiting, asymptomatic condition seen in infants and young children. Single or multiple yellow, brown or reddish papules appear. Histopathology reveals Touton giant cells, which are histiocytes loaded with lipid. Lesions almost always disappear before puberty. Usually benign, this condition has been associated with neurofibromatosis and myelogenous leukaemia.

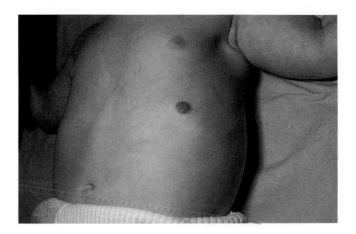

Figure 6.34 Juvenile xanthogranuloma: a 4-month-old infant with a trunk lesion.

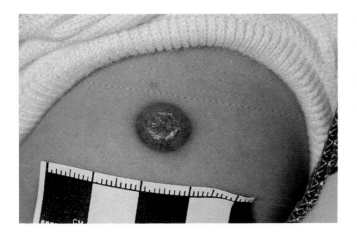

Figure 6.35 Juvenile xanthogranuloma: an uncommon giant lesion over the upper arm in a 7-month-old boy. This was excised because of its increasing size.

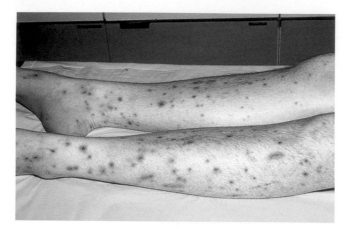

Figure 6.36 Lymphoma: a girl of 14 years old with irritant papules, some eroded, widespread and occurring particularly over the lower limbs. An initial clinical diagnosis of papular urticaria was made (Chapter 3) but she had widespread lymphadenopathy and history revealed cough, fatigue, weight loss and chest X-ray showed a mediastinal mass. She had Hodgkin's disease which responded to chemotherapy. Skin lesions showed a non-specific histology but, of course, itching was an important symptom in this child.

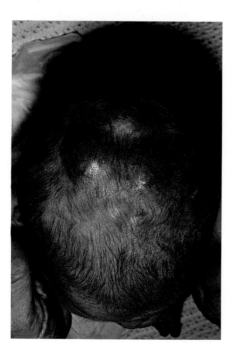

Figure 6.37 Leukaemia: a neonate with congenital purplish subcutaneous nodules which altered in size. This infant had acute monoblastic leukaemia, which has a poor prognosis, and sadly died of septicaemia despite intensive therapy.

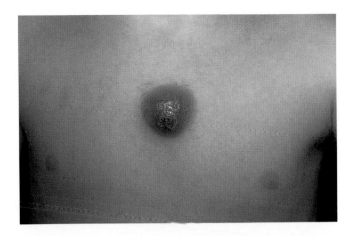

Figure 6.38
Leukaemia: a 23-month-old infant with a chest nodule due to acute myeloid leukaemia, which responded to chemotherapy. He also had smaller lesions over the scalp and shoulder. He has been in remission for more than three years.

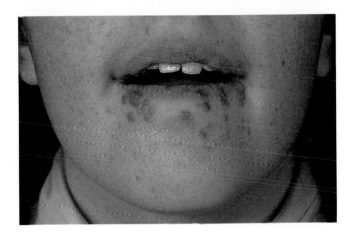

Figure 6.39
Sarcoidosis: a girl of 17 years old with brownish papules over her chin. No systemic evidence of sarcoid was found. Sarcoidosis is rare in children and tends to present with acute symptoms such as weight loss, fatigue, low-grade fever, eye changes, bone and joint pains. Sarcoid lesions are non-caseating and granulomatous on histopathological examination.

FURTHER READING

Hartley AH, Rabinowitz LG. Pediatric dermatology. *Dermatol Clin* 1997; **15**: 111–19.

7

Connective Tissue Disorders

INTRODUCTION

Hypertrophic scars in children following a scald, for instance, tend to flatten with time although this may take years and, in general, patience is the order of the day. Granuloma annulare is a rather odd benign self-limiting entity first described over a century ago. It is commonly mistaken for ringworm not responding to treatment but the lack of inflammation and scaling are important and should provide clues to diagnosis of this relatively common condition. A girl with lichen sclerosus et atrophicus, an uncommon condition, may be sent to me with a complaint of perineal itching or soreness but typical perineal pallor will be visible on examination.

Scleroderma

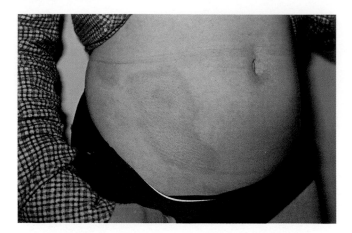

Figure 7.1 Morphoea: a large, localized patch of common morphoea over the abdomen, with small adjacent patch. Note the active edge of the main lesion. Morphoea is scleroderma localized to the skin, and it occurs in various forms. In the *common form* there is an enlarging plaque, in which the skin is firm and bound down to underlying tissues; there is usually no muscle involvement. A localized red or purplish area appears and becomes indurated. It is commonly seen on the trunk in the form of an oval-shaped area often with a violaceous zone surrounding it in active lesions. Lesions are single or few and tend to resolve spontaneously.

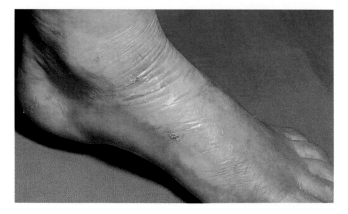

Figure 7.2 Morphoea: a girl of 5½-years old with linear morphoea. Note the binding down of the skin over the foot.

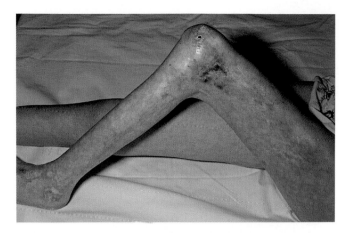

Figure 7.3 Morphoea: this shows the same child as shown in Figure 7.2 four years later. She had the rare, disabling pansclerotic form of linear morphoea with whole limb involvement, muscle involvement, limb shortening, a stiff ankle and knee contraction. Oral penicillamine did not help. A few years later the condition burnt itself out but left her with a wizened limb. Despite her infirmity she won medals for swimming at the Disabled Olympics and had a normal vaginal delivery of a baby less than ten years after this photograph was taken.

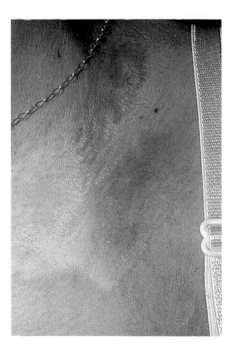

Figure 7.4 Chronic graft-versus-host disease: a girl of 17 years old with skin sclerosis over the left side of the neck. This followed a bone marrow transplant (she had acute lymphoblastic leukaemia). She had skin involvement of the upper chest and lower back also. Chronic GVHD occurs some months post-transplantation and the skin is commonly involved. The two main types of lesions are lichen planus-like or sclerodermatous. The latter are indurated sclerotic whitish–yellow plaques with a poorly defined edge and patchy hyperpigmentation may be visible.

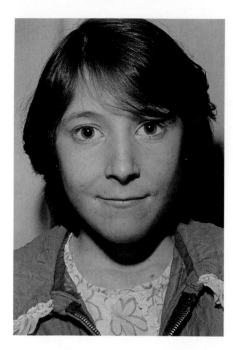

Figure 7.5 Systemic sclerosis: a girl of 13 years old with systemic sclerosis, showing a rather beaked nose. *This is a distinct entity from morphoea.* The initial manifestation is commonly Raynaud's syndrome, although weight loss and weakness may also be early symptoms. Visible skin changes begin in the fingers and can remain localized there. The fingers may be swollen initially but then the skin becomes bound down appearing shiny and there may be both hyper- and hypo-pigmentation. Later atrophic changes occur with thinning, telangiectasia and subcutaneous atrophy. Calcinosis, finger-tip ulceration, and a characteristic facies with beaked nose and puckering of mouth can also occur. Linear telangiectases over the posterior nail folds are common. It is important to assess pulmonary, bowel and renal function regularly. The course is unpredictable and spontaneous improvement can occur but renal and cardiac failure are serious complications.

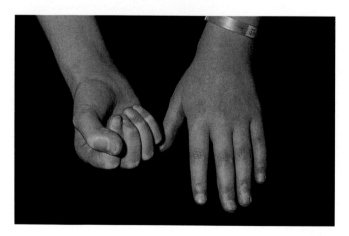

Figure 7.6 Systemic sclerosis: the same child as shown in Figure 7.5 showing binding down of the skin and restricted finger movement.

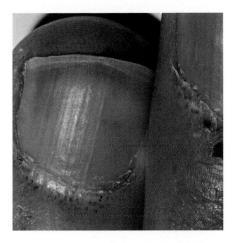

Figure 7.7 Systemic sclerosis: an adolescent male with prominent posterior nail fold telangiectases.

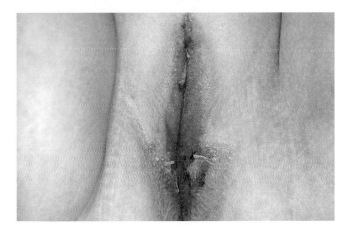

Figure 7.8 Lichen sclerosus et atrophicus: eroded perineal skin which followed blistering in a 9½-year-old child. The condition virtually resolved within three to four years of onset. Lichen sclerosus et atrophicus is a chronic inflammatory skin disorder of unknown cause. Lesions are usually smaller than those of morphoea and often involve the vulva. It can occur at any age and 90% of cases are females. Well-defined atrophic changes associated with pallor occur in the skin over the clitoris and labia minora and lesions often extend to the perianal region giving a figure-of-eight pattern. Vaginal discharge, dysuria, constipation and pruritus vulvae may be complained of in children and erythema and blistering may also be seen. Potent topical corticosteroids have a place when blistering occurs or if pruritus is marked, but many children manage their condition with emollients only. Perineal involvement in girls must not be misdiagnosed as *sexual abuse*, although, of course, the two may co-exist and the latter has been occasionally reported.

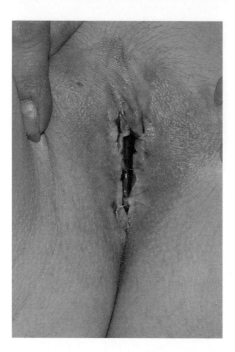

Figure 7.9 Lichen sclerosus et atrophicus: child showing eroded vulval skin with some haemorrhage.

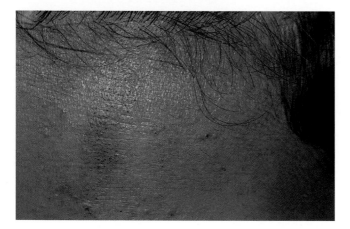

Figure 7.10 Lichen sclerosus et atrophicus: a 14-years-old boy with a bluish–white patch over his upper forehead which resolved in due course. This is an uncommon site. In boys, lichen sclerosus usually involves the foreskin resulting in an acquired *phimosis*, sometimes requiring circumcision.

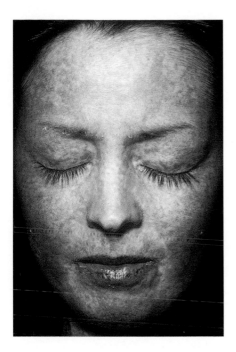

Figure 7.11 Systemic lupus erythematosus: a 20-year-old female with widespread blotchy facial erythema. She had the condition for a number of years and died of renal failure. In children and adolescents, lupus erythematosus is usually of the systemic type and resembles the adult disease. Arthritis, arthralgia, fever and skin eruptions are the most common presenting features. Facial skin eruption may appear as widespread erythema with or without oedema, erythema over the butterfly area of the face, or with time chronic discoid patches. Light-sensitivity occurs in about one-third of patients. More widespread eruption may also occur along with scalp alopecia. *Livedo reticularis*, a physical sign with many causes, which indicates capillary and venous stasis in cooled skin, may also be visible. Treatment depends on the severity of the disorder and many children respond simply to bed rest, aspirin and avoidance of sun exposure. Neonatal lupus has been mentioned in Chapter 1.

Figure 7.12 Systemic lupus erythematosus: same patient as in Figure 7.11 with blotchy erythema over back.

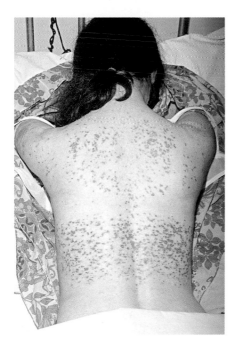

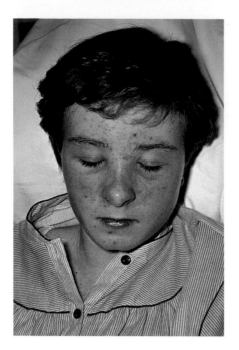

Figure 7.13 Dermatomyositis: violaceous erythema visible over the cheeks and around the eyes. This primarily affects skin and striated muscle but often involves the gastrointestinal tract also. Skin signs tend to be florid and muscle pain and tenderness marked: Any association with malignancy is rare. Girls are affected twice as frequently as boys and the mean age of onset is about seven years in children. Muscle weakness involving the proximal limb muscles (shoulder and pelvic muscles) and anterior neck muscles is the most common initial symptom. Skin eruption is violaceous and often oedematous. The face is most commonly involved, especially around the eyes, and also the upper chest, elbows, knees, knuckles and around the nails. The main pathological feature of juvenile dermatomyositis is a vasculitis affecting small arteries and veins of muscle, skin, subcutaneous tissue and bowel. Prognosis varies but many children recover completely without any specific therapy but oral corticosteroid therapy preferably in low dosage and of short duration may be necessary.

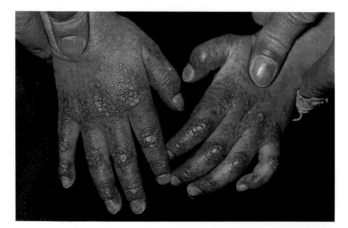

Figure 7.14 Dermatomyositis: a female infant showing striking violaceous erythema over the knuckles and skin overlying the interphalangeal joints. She never had any clinical muscle weakness, although slight elevation of muscle enzymes were found initially. She made a full recovery following short-term oral steroid therapy.

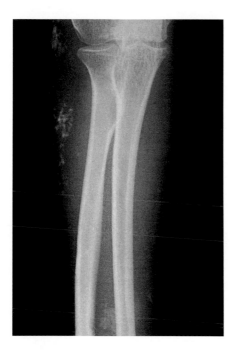

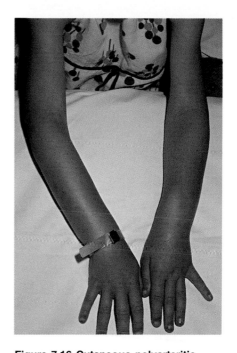

Figure 7.15 Dermatomyositis: a radiograph showing soft tissue calcification over the upper limb. *Calcinosis* develops more commonly in children than in adults and deposits, which are usually subcutaneous, may often ulcerate and discharge.

Figure 7.16 Cutaneous polyarteritis nodosa: the forearms and back of the left hand are swollen in this 5-year-old girl. Marked livedo was visible over the arms 5 months later when she was much better, the swelling having subsided. This illustrates the benign cutaneous form of polyarteritis nodosa which affects the skin, skeletal muscles, and peripheral nerves or skin only. It presents as nodules generally on the lower legs, and these nodules are often very tender. Many resolve but ulceration can occur and some ulcers may be necrotic. Nodules are associated with livedo reticularis and histopathology reveals a necrotizing vasculitis at the junction of dermis and subcutaneous tissue.

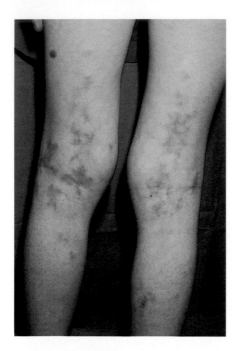

Figure 7.17 Cutaneous polyarteritis nodosa: livedo reticularis with nodulation in the same child as shown in Figure 7.16. Nodules were palpable both adjacent to and in the areas of livedo.

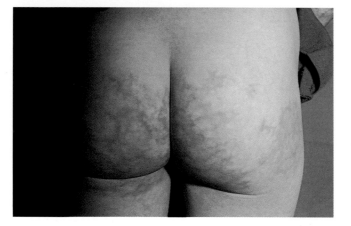

Figure 7.18 Cutaneous polyarteritis nodosa: persistent cyanotic mottled discoloration of livedo reticularis visible over the buttocks in the same child as shown in Figures 7.16 and 7.17. She is now in her mid-twenties and is still subject to recurrent bouts of cutaneous polyarteritis nodosa but her disease remains confined to the skin.

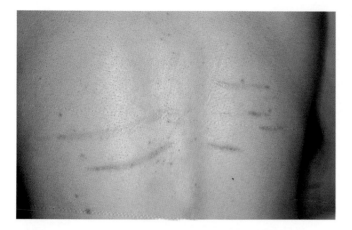

Figure 7.19 Striae atrophicae: illustrated are recently-appearing transverse lesions which will flatten and become less obvious in time. They are a common, normal finding at puberty and later, whether the individual is thin or obese. They may first develop soon after the appearance of pubic hair. Commonest sites are the lumbosacral region and the outer thighs in boys, and the thighs, buttocks and breasts in girls. At first pink, raised and weal-like, they soon become flat, smooth and bluish in colour. They tend to be linear and become less noticeable with increasing age.

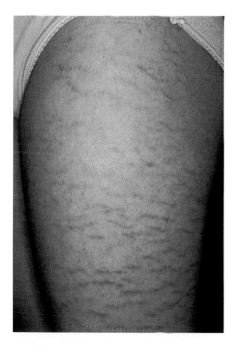

Figure 7.20 Striae atrophicae: striae over the thigh in a girl of 12-years-old.

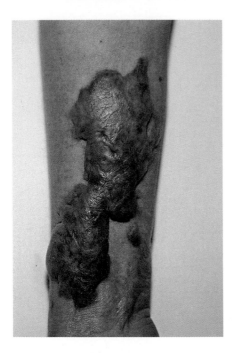

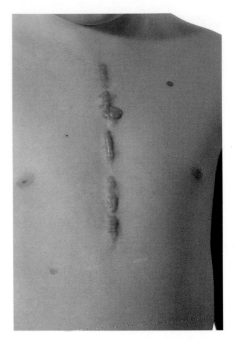

Figure 7.21 Hypertrophic scar: the forearm in this boy of 8-years-old was scalded by steam from a kettle 6 months previously. There was visible flattening of the scar 6 months after this photo was taken and further improvement occurred. Hypertrophic scars in response to injury tend to stay within the margin of the trauma lesion. Although fresh scars in children are often hypertrophic, with passage of time and patience, they often contract and become less apparent. It is important to mention the above to parents, for often the most unsightly scars flatten spontaneously within a few years. A *keloid* is a benign well-demarcated area of fibrous tissue overgrowth that extends beyond the original defect. Like a hypertrophic scar, a keloid is a response to an injury that may sometimes be trivial. It tends to increase in size long after healing has taken place. Afro-Caribbeans are more prone to develop keloids.

Figure 7.22 Hypertrophic scar: chest scar in a 3-year-old child. He had cardiac surgery two years previously but the scar persisted. Hypertrophic scars over the chest have a tendency to be more persistent than those over limbs.

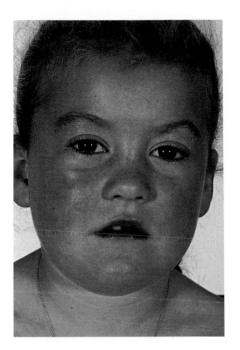

Figure 7.23 Scleroedema: a 6-year-old girl with fixed facial expression. Tight skin develops over the face and elsewhere in this uncommon condition, which may be preceded by an infection. It usually begins over the back, neck or face with symmetrical tightness of the skin. It tends to resolve spontaneously within two years, as in the child shown, but it is sometimes associated with diabetes and in such patients the disease may be of longer duration.

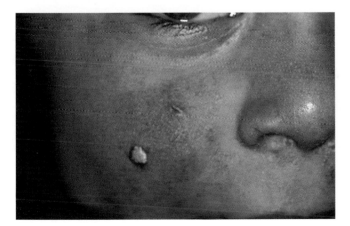

Figure 7.24 Calcinosis cutis: a 2-year-old boy with a solitary lesion on the cheek, said to have been present at birth. Calcinosis cutis can be either localized or widespread, and of unknown cause or secondary to metabolic disorders, or to tissue damage as in connective tissue disorders such as dermatomyositis (Figure 7.15).

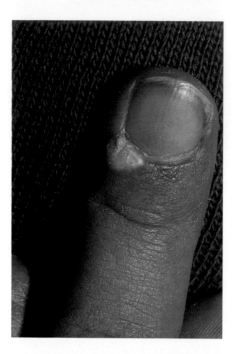

Figure 7.25 Calcinosis cutis: a 4-year-old boy with long-standing calcium deposition over one of two affected fingers. He was well otherwise.

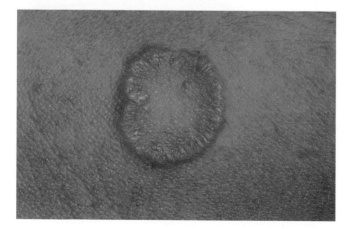

Figure 7.26 Granuloma annulare: a ringed lesion with a raised non-scaling edge. This may occur anywhere but usually over bony prominences and especially over the hands and feet. Children and young adults are most commonly affected and it is more common in females. Early lesions begin as smooth flesh-coloured papules that slowly undergo central involution and peripheral extension to form oval or irregular rings with elevated, often beaded borders. Lesions may be single or multiple and are usually 1–3 cm in diameter, but more extensive patches sometimes with a violaceous hue may occur. Deeper *subcutaneous* lesions over the shins, for instance, may also occur. The lesions tend to disappear spontaneously.

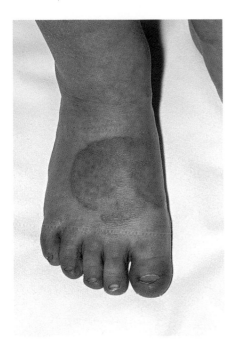

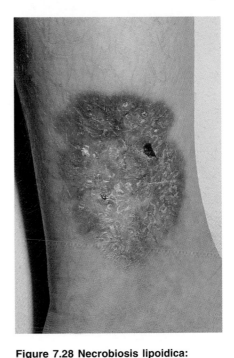

Figure 7.27 Granuloma annulare: a violaceous, extending, asymptomatic patch over the dorsum of the foot. Note the lack of inflammation and scaling.

Figure 7.28 Necrobiosis lipoidica: close-up of the leg In a diabetic girl of 15-years-old with the outer portion of the lesion showing telangiectasia and a yellowish colour. This degenerative disorder of dermal connective tissue may appear at any age and occurs in 0.3% of diabetics, sometimes preceding the onset of diabetes. It occurs in non-diabetics also. Lesions are most common over the pretibial area, beginning as an erythematous patch which gradually enlarges and develops slowly into a brownish–yellow sclerotic plaque. The centre of a plaque is often atrophic with a translucent surface. Lesions are often best left untreated but early lesions can sometimes be aborted with intralesional triamcinolone acetonide.

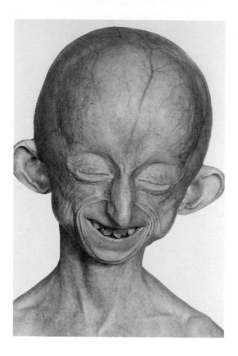

Figure 7.29 Progeria: a boy of 12-years-old showing the striking premature ageing appearance. In this rare disorder there is premature and rapid ageing with an onset in infancy. Patients develop atherosclerosis and die of cardiac or cerebral vascular disease usually in their early teens.

FURTHER READING

Ginarte M, Pereiro M, Toribio J. Cutaneous polyarteritis nodosa in a child. *Pediat Dermatol* 1998; **15**: 103–7.
Ridley CM. Genital lichen sclerosus (lichen sclerosus et atrophicus) in childhood and adolescence. *J Roy S Med* 1993; **86**: 69–75.

8

Vascular Disorders and Drug Eruptions

INTRODUCTION

Chilblains are uncommon these days with modern heating. In any case, affected children would not usually require referral to a clinic. Acute urticaria is common and will usually be managed by the Family Practitioner but chronic urticaria is frequently seen in my clinics. Prick testing in young children with chronic urticaria is unrewarding as the results are unreliable, and even in older children testing is often unhelpful. Taking a good history is essential in patients with urticaria. Drug eruptions are seen from time to time but do not present a common problem in children.

Urticaria

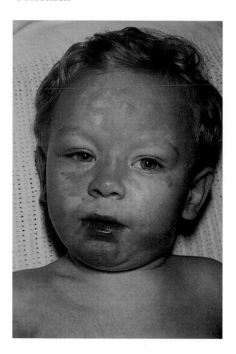

Figure 8.1 Ordinary urticaria: patchy erythema and wealing over the face is shown. Ordinary urticaria or hives is an itchy erythematous eruption characterized by flesh-coloured weals. It is due to a local increased permeability of capillaries and small venules. It may be associated with *angioedema* in which swelling of the lips, eyelids, genitalia, tongue or larynx can occur. *Giant urticaria* indicates widespread areas of skin involvement. Ordinary urticaria is very common and important causes are drugs, food, inhalants or infections, although many cases are of unknown cause. Acute attacks respond to oral antihistamines and angioedema usually responds also, but if threatening the airway intramuscular adrenaline injection 1 in 1000 is indicated, dosage depending on age and weight, and this can be followed, if required, by intravenous or intramuscular hydrocortisone.

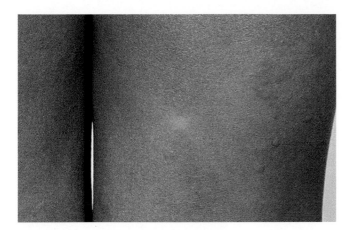

Figure 8.2 Ordinary urticaria: a boy of 7-years-old with weals over the thigh.

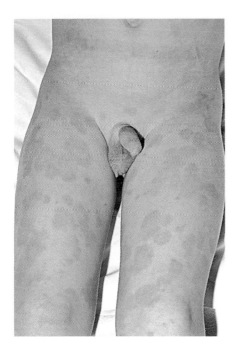

Figure 8.3 Ordinary urticaria: a boy of 8-years-old with urticaria, thought to be drug-induced, with some purpura over the scrotum. It is not uncommon for some urticarial lesions to show a purpuric element.

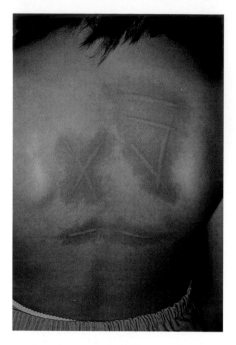

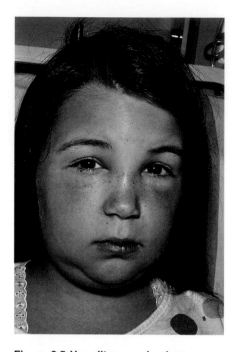

Figure 8.4 Dermographism (factitious urticaria): this picture shows the form of *physical urticaria* induced by trauma in a 10-year-old girl. Of the physical urticarias, dermographism (factitious urticaria) indicates wealing that occurs after the skin is firmly stroked or rubbed. This physical urticaria is seen in at least 5% of normal people, and may or may not be symptomatic. It may begin in childhood and can give rise to much itching. The wealing tendency with light trauma persists for months or years. There are many other types of *physical urticaria*, for example those due to *cold, heat, sun or water* and *cholinergic urticaria* where weals are small and attacks are precipitated by exercise, heat and emotional stress. Dermographism may also be elicited in *mastocytoses* (see Chapter 10).

Figure 8.5 Hereditary angioedema: a 12-year-old girl who was admitted to hospital being unable to swallow. She improved rapidly with conservative treatment. There was a family history, and affected members tended to improve with age. This is a rare, autosomal dominant condition due to reduced or inactive C1 esterase inhibitor. It usually starts in early childhood and presents with subcutaneous swellings often accompanied by abdominal pain. There is no urticaria. Attacks are often precipitated by trauma. The danger in some families is of laryngeal obstruction due to oedema. Infusion of fresh frozen plasma is effective in severe acute attacks but purified C1 inhibitor preparation is also available.

Erythema

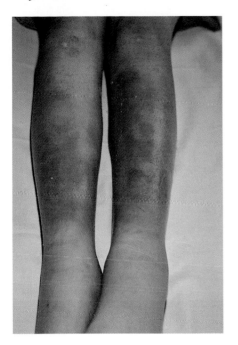

Figure 8.6 Erythema nodosum: a girl of 11 years old with tender nodules over her legs. Nodules were discrete at first becoming confluent. Note the ankle swelling. This presents with discrete, painful, red nodules, which may become confluent over shins. Streptococcal infections and, much less commonly, primary tuberculosis infection, are well known causes. No cause at all is found in about 30% of patients. Lesions may also occur over the thighs, arms and even over the face. Attacks last 3–6 weeks and the nodules leave bruise-like discolouration as they resolve. The nodules do not ulcerate.

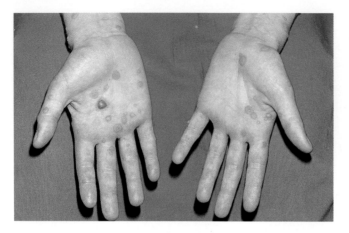

Figure 8.7 Erythema multiforme: typical target lesions over the palms with a haemorrhagic blister over the right palm. This is an inflammatory condition which affects skin and mucous membranes. It often occurs without obvious cause but it has many causes. Herpes simplex and mycoplasma are well known precipitating factors but drugs are not usually an important cause in children. Following herpes simplex, erythema multiforme may appear 1–2 weeks later. The target or iris lesion is typical, consisting of a purple centre which may blister, surrounded by an erythematous ring. Lesions occur over the hands, feet, elbows and knees and there may be painful ulcers over the buccal mucosa and in more severe cases, other mucosae. The condition can be subdivided into minor and major forms. Mouth washes and oral antihistamines are routine for minor erythema multiforme. Systemic and topical aciclovir commenced early in a simplex attack may prevent erythema multiforme occurring in those with frequent recurrent simplex-precipitated erythema multiforme. *Stevens-Johnson syndrome* is a severe, bullous major form with atypical skin lesions in which drug sensitivity as a cause does seem more important than virus infection.

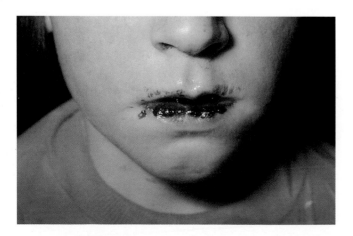

Figure 8.8 Erythema multiforme: a lip ulceration in a boy with recent mycoplasma infection.

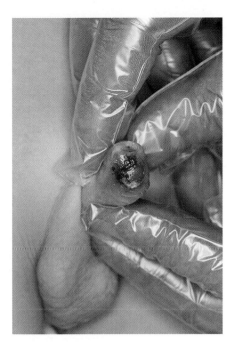

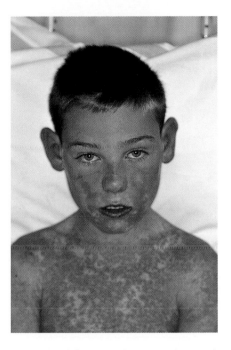

Figure 8.9 Erythema multiforme: the same boy as shown in Figure 8.8 with penile ulceration. He had few skin lesions.

Figure 8.10 Toxic erythema: widespread morbilliform erythema in a 10-year-old child, likely due to a viral sore throat. This is a term sometimes used to describe scarlatiniform or morbilliform eruptions due to drugs, viral or bacterial infections or of unknown cause. Morbilliform eruptions are usually due to virus infections and drugs. The scarlatiniform eruption may be widespread or localized to the palms and soles and spontaneous resolution usually followed by desquamation occurs in 2–3 weeks. Exotoxins of haemolytic streptococcus (and rarely staphylococcus) and drugs are known causes.

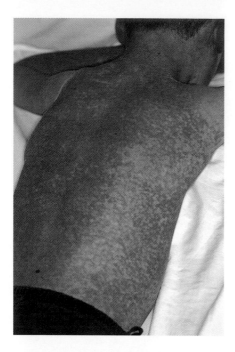

Figure 8.11 Toxic erythema: the same boy as shown in Figure 8.10 with extensive morbilliform eruption over his back.

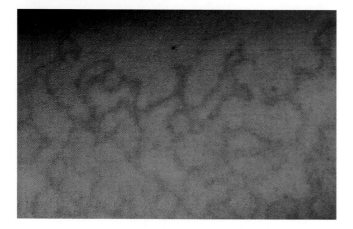

Figure 8.12 Erythema marginatum: the reticulated pattern is shown. This erythema is probably specific for active rheumatic fever and is asymptomatic. It has become rare in the developed world with the decline of rheumatic fever. It first appears over the trunk and consists of flat or slightly raised rings which may be discrete or by enlargement produce a reticulated pattern. Characteristically, lesions fade within a few hours to a few days. Recurrent crops can appear at intervals for weeks.

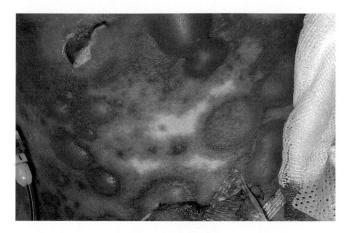

Figure 8.13 Toxic epidermal necrolysis: a boy of 3 years old showing erythema, bullae and separation of the skin over the trunk. He was treated in the intensive care unit. He began with an upper respiratory infection and then mild erythema multiforme but he gradually deteriorated as illustrated. Virus infection was the probable primary cause. Toxic epidermal necrolysis is a serious condition affecting all age groups and it may be due to drugs, infections or other causes. Mucosal involvement is usual, with the oropharynx, eyes and genitalia particularly affected. The site of skin separation is the epidermo-dermal junction and there is epithelial cell necrosis. Treatment depends on the cause and is as for a burn, usually in a special unit. Duration may be weeks and there is a mortality of 25% or more. The boundary between severe Stevens–Johnson syndrome and toxic epidermal necrolysis is often unclear.

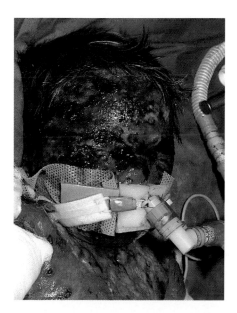

Figure 8.14 Toxic epidermal necrolysis: the same boy as shown in Figure 8.13 showing progressive disease with crusting over the face, and chest, and marked erythema. He made a remarkable recovery after several months, despite many complications.

Purpura

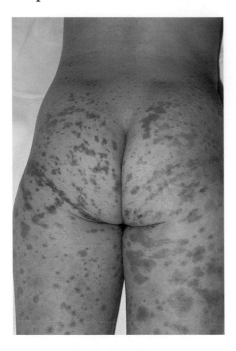 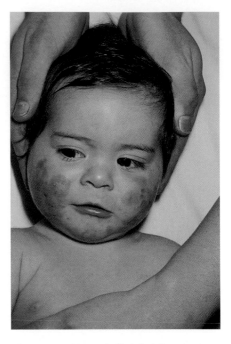

Figure 8.15 Henoch–Schönlein purpura: a girl of 11 years old with purpura over the buttocks and lower limbs. This is an *allergic vasculitis* and the most common childhood vasculitis. In about one-third of patients an upper respiratory tract infection precedes the eruption. Purpura, some of which is palpable, occurs predominantly over the lower limbs and buttocks and may be associated with joint pains or with abdominal and renal complications. There may be limb oedema and this is not necessarily in purpuric areas. Abdominal symptoms due to vasculitis of gastrointestinal vessels present most commonly as colic. Renal involvement is usually just a transient microscopic haematuria and the condition usually settles over a few weeks. However, glomerulonephritis can occur as a complication. Systemic steroids are only useful in the presence of severe abdominal pain.

Figure 8.16 Henoch–Schönlein purpura: facial lesions are not uncommon, as seen in this 6-month-old Venezuelan infant.

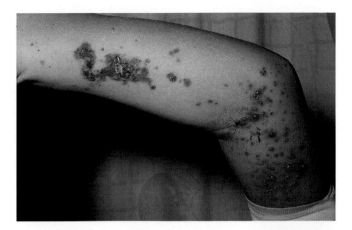

Figure 8.17 Henoch–Schönlein purpura: blisters and purpura in an 8-year-old child. Visible blisters are very uncommon in this disorder.

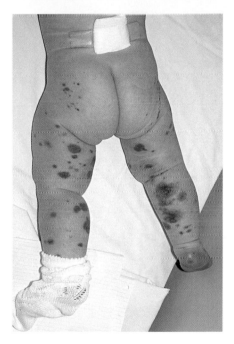

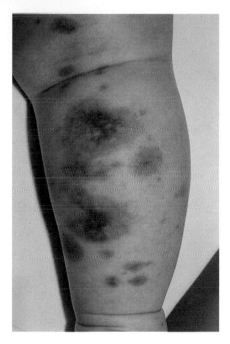

Figure 8.18 Acute haemorrhagic oedema of infancy: typical purpuric lesions over the legs. This rare entity seems to be distinct from Henoch–Schönlein purpura. For instance, it occurs in a younger age group (infants between 4 months and 2 years), spontaneous resolution occurs within 1–3 weeks and visceral involvement is very uncommon. Inflammatory oedema and purpura occur over the limbs and face and lesions over the limbs are often medallion-like.

Figure 8.19 Acute haemorrhagic oedema of infancy: close-up of the right calf of the infant shown in Figure 8.18 showing medallion-like lesions.

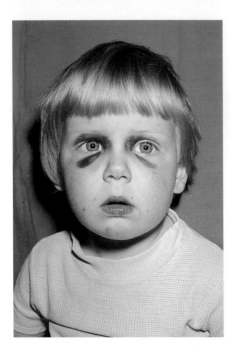

Figure 8.20 Immune thrombocytopenic purpura: differential diagnosis would include non-accidental injury. ITP often occurs after a viral infection, particularly rubella. Bleeding occurs into the skin and may occur in any organ. The majority of patients recover spontaneously within a few months.

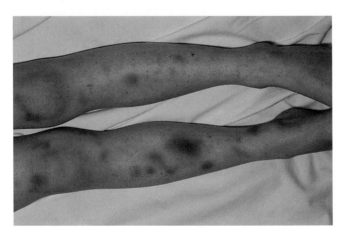

Figure 8.21 Immune thrombocytopenic purpura: purpura over the legs in a 6-year-old child. It followed varicella in this child.

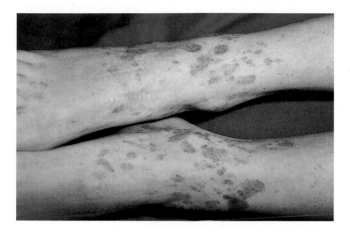

Figure 8.22 Pigmented purpuric dermatosis: this girl of 12
years old had itching purpura with the involvement of lower
limbs and buttocks and slight upper-limb involvement.
Asymptomatic or slightly irritant dark red or brown purpuric
patches with haemosiderin staining appear over the lower legs
particularly. Histopathology is of lymphocytic vasculitis. The
condition may persist for years but some cases do resolve.

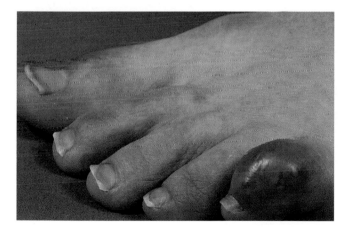

Figure 8.23 Chilblains: florid chilblains of the little toe in this
13-year-old girl. Chilblains (perniosis) are localized, inflammatory
lesions that arise as an abnormal reaction to cold and are
particularly seen in homes lacking central heating. They occur
on the fingers, toes, thighs, nose and ears. They appear
cyanotic and can ulcerate. They may occur over local
accumulations of fat such as the *wrists of infants* where swelling
and coldness will be present. Treatment is warm clothing and
adequate home heating.

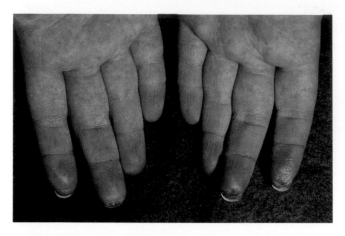

Figure 8.24 Raynaud's syndrome: a girl of 7 years old with cyanotic fingertips. She has improved with increasing age. In this syndrome there is peripheral vascular disturbance with spasm of the digital arteries producing numbness, tingling, burning and colour changes. A typical attack consists of pallor of one or more fingers, followed by cyanosis and then erythema. There may be no apparent cause but the condition may also be part of systemic sclerosis or other conditions such as occlusive arterial disease or a cervical rib.

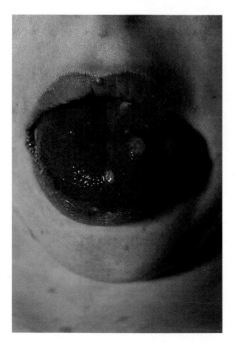

Figure 8.25 Kawasaki disease: a boy of 5 years old with an inflamed red tongue. The tongue also shows ulceration but this was due to concurrent varicella. He had other features of Kawasaki disease including cardiac involvement. This is also called the mucocutaneous lymph node syndrome and is an acute febrile illness of unknown aetiology that produces a multisystem vasculitis. Persistent fever, non-specific skin eruption, erythema and/or oedema of hands and feet, inflammation of mucous membranes, conjunctivitis and cervical lymphadenopathy are usual.

Drug eruptions

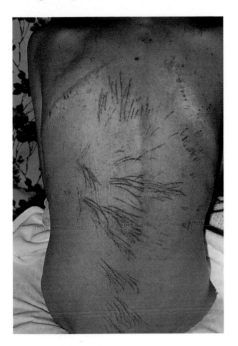

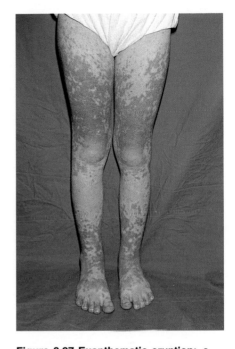

Figure 8.26 Pruritus: severe itching and scratch marks in a girl of 15 years old. This preceded an exanthematic eruption due to a diuretic prescribed in high dosage for cardiac failure. It should be remembered that pruritus may precede a drug eruption.

Figure 8.27 Exanthematic eruption: a girl of 6 years old with florid exanthem most marked over the limbs. She had received various antibiotics and ampicillin was considered the most likely cause. This term indicates a widespread erythematous maculopapular eruption which may be morbilliform. Ampicillin eruptions are usually exanthematic and appear 5–14 days after starting treatment.

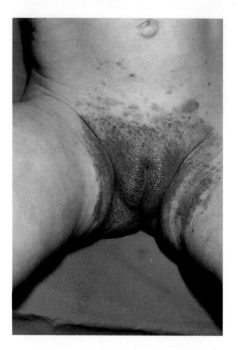

Figure 8.28 Topical corticosteroid-induced eruption: erythema in a napkin eruption due to, or worsened by, frequent application of a potent corticosteroid. *Topical steroids,* particularly the more potent ones, can give rise to skin atrophy which is usually reversible and to striae which are usually irreversible. Application, particularly under occlusion, enhances steroid damage and absorption. Note that disposable nappies are occlusive. Even prolonged use of the mildly potent hydrocortisone itself over widespread areas of skin should not be encouraged. Excessive *growth of hair* is occasionally seen at the site of prolonged steroid application and *infection* is not an uncommon side-effect in view of the lowered resistance produced by steroid inhibition of the normal inflammatory response. Repeated applications of potent and usually fluorinated steroids, particularly under occlusion and when used long-term, may lead to interference with *pituitary–adrenal function* and *retard growth.*

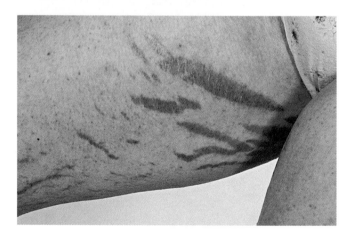

Figure 8.29 Topical corticosteroid-induced eruption: a 20-year-old girl with widespread striae over the thighs. She had used a very potent topical steroid for 1 year, mainly over hands and feet.

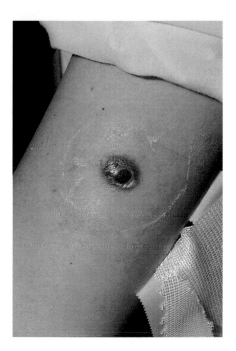

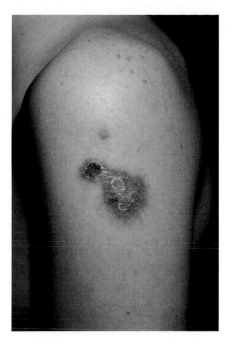

Figure 8.30 Bacillus Calmette-Guérin (BCG) vaccine: superficial ulceration 4–5 months after inoculation in a boy of 12 years old. No bacterial growth was evident from swab culture. Such ulcers usually heal spontaneously but saline cleansing may be helpful. 3% oxytetracycline ointment (or cream) for persistent ulceration may be prescribed. *Ulcers* and *abscesses* may follow too-deep injection of BCG vaccine. *Hypertrophic* and *keloid scars* may develop after prolonged site infection. *Granulomata*, including lupus vulgaris (Figure 8.31), also occur.

Figure 8.31 Bacillus Calmette-Guérin (BCG) vaccine: this 14-year-old boy developed lupus vulgaris at the injection site 6 months after vaccination. Such reactions usually heal spontaneously, but application of oxytetracycline ointment/cream and/or oral erythromycin for 2–4 months is usually effective.

FURTHER READING

Becker DS. Toxic epidermal necrolysis *Lancet* 1998; **351**: 1417–20.

Gonggryp LA, Todd G. Acute hemorrhagic edema of Childhood (AHE) *Pediatr Dermatol* 1998; **15**: 426–28.

Nussinovitch M, Prais D, Finkelstein Y, Varsano I. Cutaneous manifestations of Henoch-Schönlein Purpura in young children *Pediatr Dermatol* 1998; **15**: 426–28.

9

Genodermatoses

CONTENTS

INTRODUCTION

Varying degrees of ichthyosis vulgaris are commonly seen as an associated finding in children presenting with atopic dermatitis, and it is the most common of the ichthyoses. Neurofibromatosis (NF-1) is not always recognized, even with florid signs, but multiple café-au-lait patches often alert the doctor to consider it in the differential diagnosis of such patches. Some genodermatoses are considered in Chapters 1, 5, 10 and elsewhere.

Autosomal dominant

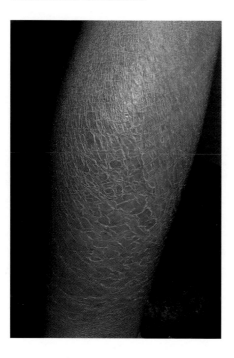

Figure 9.1 Ichthyosis vulgaris: a 5½-year-old boy with scaling skin. This is the most common of the many ichthyoses (see Chapter 1) with a reported incidence of 1 in 250 in the English population. Small, white scales appear during early childhood; however, shin scales are often large. Cubital and popliteal fossae are characteristically spared. Accentuated palmar and plantar skin markings are common. It is often seen in association with *atopic dermatitis*.

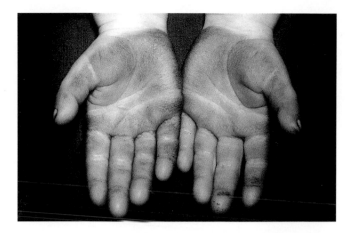

Figure 9.2 Hereditary palmoplantar keratoderma: the change from normal to affected skin is well-defined. This was an isolated, harmless, inherited abnormality appearing in infancy in this child's family. There are many skin disorders in which palmoplantar keratoderma occurs or it may be an isolated finding.

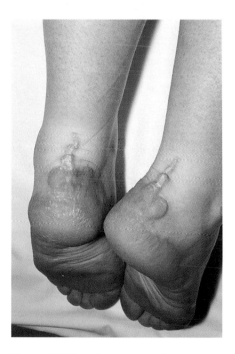

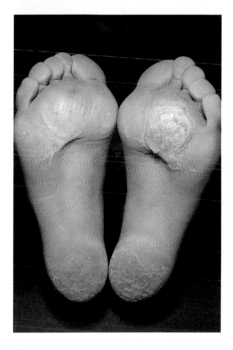

Figure 9.3 Hereditary palmoplantar keratoderma: a girl of 11 years old with thickened skin over the soles, which first appeared in infancy and extended to achilles skin in a starfish pattern. There was an association of keratoderma with deafness in the family.

Figure 9.4 Hereditary palmoplantar keratoderma: a boy with thickened skin localized to weight-bearing areas of the soles. There was a family history of oesophageal carcinoma. There is a *rare association* (described in two families in Liverpool, UK) between hereditary palmoplantar keratoderma usually appearing after infancy, oral preleukoplakia and/or leukoplakia and development of oesophageal carcinoma in later adult life.

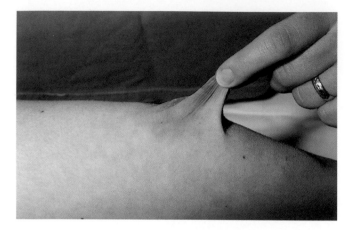

Figure 9.5 Ehlers–Danlos syndrome (EDS): this picture demonstrates hyperextensibility of skin. This syndrome has ten clinically and genetically distinct varieties, all having abnormalities of collagen. The most common types (EDS I, II and III) are autosomal dominant. Joints are easily dislocated and ligaments lax. Typical features of EDS are hyperextensibility and fragility of the skin with an increased susceptibility to bruising and hypermobility of the joints.

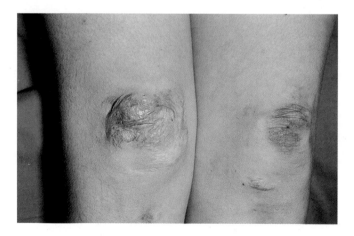

Figure 9.6 Ehlers–Danlos syndrome: unsightly, diffuse, atrophic, gaping scars over the knees.

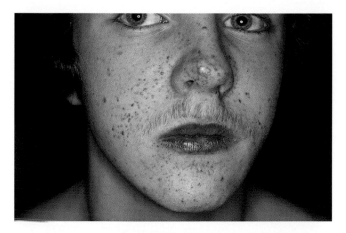

Figure 9.7 Tuberous sclerosis: facial angiofibromas are visible. Such lesions used to be incorrectly termed adenoma sebaceum. Tuberous sclerosis gives rise to angiofibromas which usually appear towards the end of the first decade as small red–brown papules on the nose and nasolabial folds. Other characteristic lesions are fibromas of the nail fold (which can be mistaken for viral warts), irregularly coarsened skin over the sacrum or nearby (shagreen patch), and small oval hypopigmented areas (ash leaf macules, which are more prominent under Wood's ultraviolet light) which are usually the earliest skin sign and may present in the neonate. A smooth red or yellow plaque over the forehead may also be an early sign of the condition. Epilepsy is an important manifestation of this disorder.

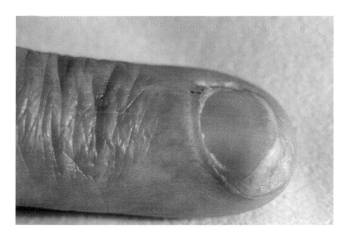

Figure 9.8 Tuberous sclerosis: subungual *fibroma* of the index finger. Such lesions do not appear before the second decade, as in this patient.

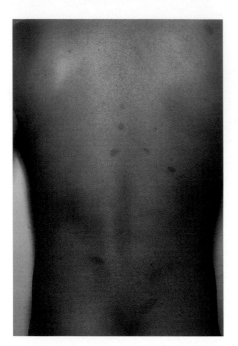

Figure 9.9 Neurofibromatosis (NF-1): Multiple café-au-lait patches are visible in this 3-year-old child. Neurofibromatosis (NF-1), which has a prevalence of about 1 in 3000 births, usually manifests as multiple benign tumours of neural tissue and multiple café-au-lait patches (six or more 1.5 cm or greater in diameter after puberty are virtually diagnostic). The patches usually develop within the first year of life and may be present at birth but the cutaneous neurofibromas do not develop until late childhood. Bilateral axillary or inguinal freckling, if present, is pathognomonic of the condition. *Lisch nodules* (pigmented iris hamartomas) are common and help to confirm the diagnosis of NF-1. Genetic counselling as in other genodermatoses, is important.

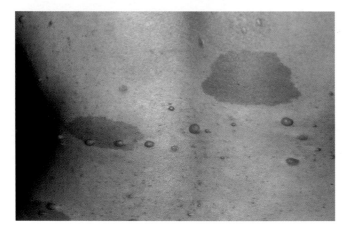

Figure 9.10 Neurofibromatosis (NF-1): large café-au-lait patches and neurofibromas are seen. Soft tumours can give the impression of being pushed through a button-hole skin defect.

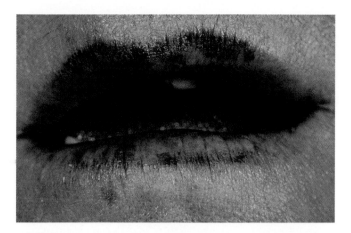

Figure 9.11 Peutz–Jeghers syndrome: characteristic pigmented spots over the lips. Pigmented macules (lentigines) usually appear in infancy or early childhood most commonly in the mouth and on and around the lips, but often also over the hands and feet. Polyposis of the small and/or large bowel is part of the syndrome and lesions are usually benign but there is a slightly increased risk of gastrointestinal carcinoma. Polyps can bleed leading to anaemia and they can also cause intussusception.

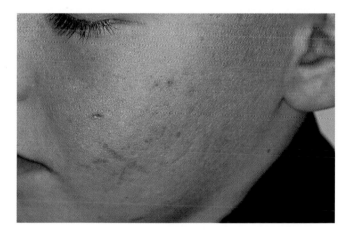

Figure 9.12 Erythropoietic protoporphyria: a young boy who presented with light intolerance. He showed striking, typical scars over the cheeks. An uncommon condition presenting as photosensitivity often by the age of 2 years. Burning or tingling of the face and hands occur after exposure to sunlight (in the UVA and longer visible light range) and serous crusts may form on the nose; bright windy days are often troublesome. There is an increased incidence of gallstones. Transient fluorescence of red blood cells is diagnostic. Oral β-carotene in the brighter weather is helpful in many affected individuals as it was in this boy.

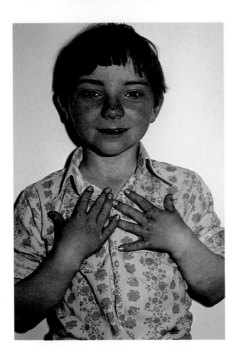

Figure 9.13 Erythropoietic protoporphyria: a boy with lesions over the nose and knuckles which left characteristic scars. He described the tingling of his hands in the sun as 'like lemonade fizzing'.

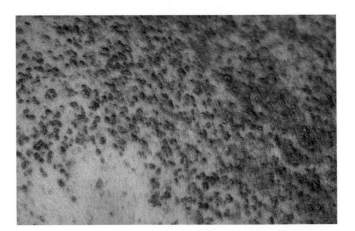

Figure 9.14 Darier's disease (keratosis follicularis): close-up of the right anterior shoulder lesions which were brown, papular and slightly scaling. A peculiar skin condition which commonly appears at puberty and is worse in warm weather, in which distinctive warty, greasy, crusted papules occur over the trunk, face, scalp and flexures. White papules may occur on the palate, and nail changes include longitudinal white or dark streaks. The palms and soles may show minute pits interrupting epidermal ridges.

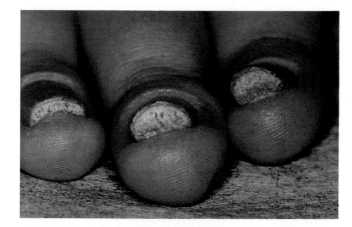

Figure 9.15 Pachyonychia congenita: a 9-year-old girl with striking abnormal thickened finger-nails. Abnormal nails are present at birth and they develop wedge-like thickening with exaggeration of the transverse curvature. Palmar and plantar hyperkeratosis occurs, followed frequently by oral leukoplakia in late childhood.

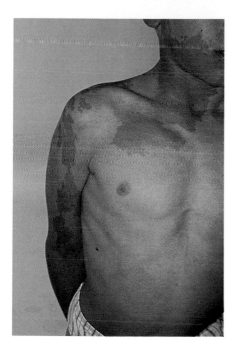

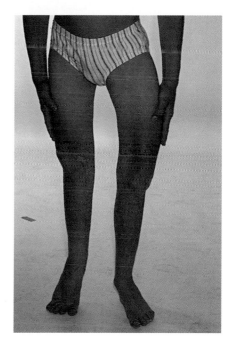

Figure 9.16 Polyostotic fibrous dysplasia (McCune–Albright syndrome): an 11-year-old boy showing patchy hyperpigmentation over the neck, shoulders and right upper limb. Cutaneous pigmentation usually develops by the age of 2 in this condition in which there is fibrous dysplasia. Precocious puberty may occur in girls. Bone lesions are associated with pain, pathological fractures and deformities.

Figure 9.17 Polyostotic fibrous dysplasia: the same child as shown in Figure 9.16 showing a thigh deformity.

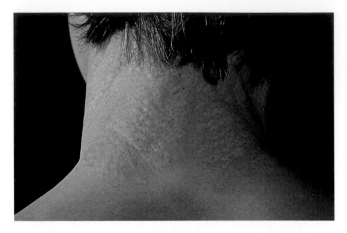

Figure 9.18 Pseudoxanthoma elasticum: plucked chicken or crêpe bandage-like skin over the back of the neck. This is a generalized connective-tissue disorder which may be dominant or recessive. It does not usually manifest until the second decade or later. The skin, eyes and cardiovascular system are affected but disease severity varies. Yellow, oval papules over the neck, axillae, cubital fossae and inguinal and periumbilical areas occur.

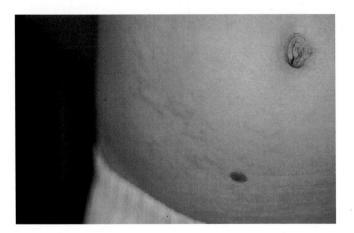

Figure 9.19 Buschke–Ollendorff syndrome: asymptomatic, yellowish, soft plaques over the abdomen in an 8½-year-old boy. This benign condition without either ocular changes or cardiovascular involvement should not be confused with pseudoxanthoma elasticum. It consists of connective tissue naevi involving the skin and *osteopoikilosis* (*spotted bones*). The skin lesions are creamy yellow soft patches.

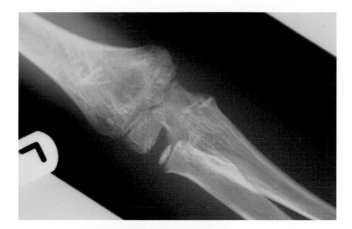

**Figure 9.20
Buschke–Ollendorff
syndrome:** a
radiograph of the left
arm of the same boy
shown in Figure 9.19
showing osteo-
poikilosis in lower
humerus particularly.

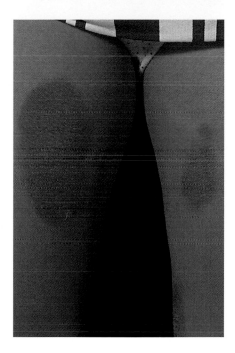

Figure 9.21 Erythrokeratoderma: a girl of
7 years old with symmetrical, well defined,
hyperpigmented patches over the thighs.
Symmetrical persistent hyperkeratotic and
hyperpigmented circumscribed patches occur
in this rare disorder. There is also a form in
which an erythematous migrating eruption
occurs.

Autosomal recessive

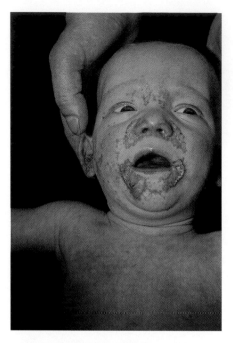 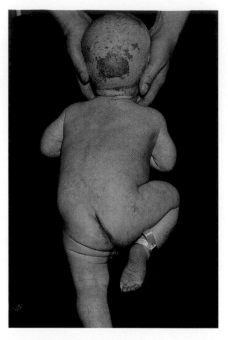

Figure 9.22 Acrodermatitis enteropathica: moist typical perioral eruption in a 4-month-old baby. Acrodermatitis enteropathica is usually seen in breast-fed infants at the time of weaning, but may also appear later. Exudative eczematous lesions with a tendency to secondary infection appear around orifices and over the scalp, hands and feet. There is diarrhoea, weight loss, irritability and hair loss from the scalp, eyebrows and eyelashes. A defect in zinc absorption is present and oral zinc sulphate effectively relieves the condition. Improvement will usually be seen within a week of therapy. Sometimes the condition improves with increasing age so that zinc can be discontinued. *Zinc deficiency* can also be an acquired disorder resulting from inadequate dietary intake or increased zinc loss. Also premature infants are often zinc deficient. Even in the breast-fed infant, despite normal maternal serum zinc levels, zinc deficiency can occur due to abnormal zinc uptake by the breast, or defective zinc secretion by the breast.

Figure 9.23 Acrodermatitis enteropathica: the same infant as shown in Figure 9.22 illustrating involvement of posterior scalp and natal cleft.

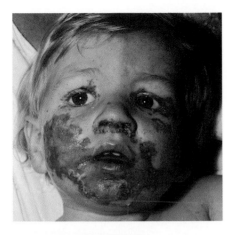

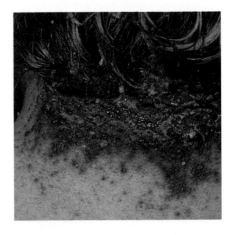

Figure 9.24 Acrodermatitis enteropathica: an 18-month-old infant with extensive perioral and nasal crusting eruption.

Figure 9.25 Acrodermatitis enteropathica: the same infant as shown in Figure 9.24 with crusting over the back of the neck.

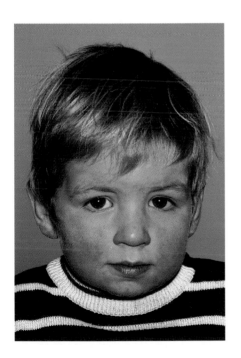

Figure 9.26 Acrodermatitis enteropathica: the same boy as in Figures 9.24 and 9.25 at the age of 2 years old and very well: now more than 5 years old, he remains on oral zinc sulphate.

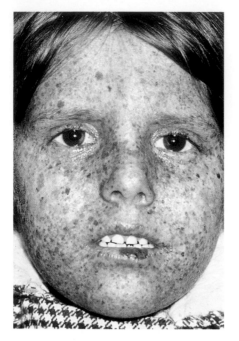

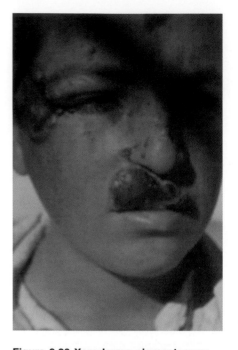

Figure 9.27 Xeroderma pigmentosum: Patchy pigmented lesions and solar keratoses over the face and an eroded lower lip. This indicates a group of rare conditions characterized by hypersensitivity to ultraviolet rays followed eventually by the development of multiple tumours including solar keratoses (benign), basal and squamous-cell carcinomas and malignant melanomas, in the exposed areas. Photosensitivity may be apparent from the age of 2 months, and erythema, which can be striking, occurs over exposed areas, particularly the face. After a few years of exposure the skin becomes dry, with freckles, hyperpigmentation, atrophy and scarring.

Figure 9.28 Xeroderma pigmentosum: an Iranian boy of 12 years old with squamous cell carcinoma above the lip, and another one lateral to the right eye. He had already lost the left eye following squamous carcinoma infiltrating the orbit. Patients may die in childhood from tumour metastases but with modern health education including the use of sunscreens, prognosis is better. The cause is a defect of the normal repair system of DNA damaged by ultraviolet rays. The condition can be identified pre-natally.

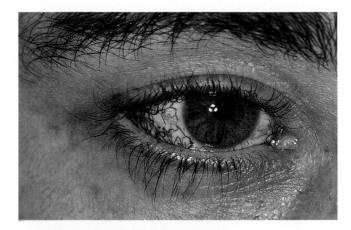

Figure 9.29 Ataxia-telangiectasia (Louis–Bar syndrome): profuse vessels over the conjunctiva are visible. This is a syndrome in which telangiectases, progressive cerebellar ataxia and recurrent respiratory infections occur. Ataxia is progressive in childhood and mental deterioration may be seen.

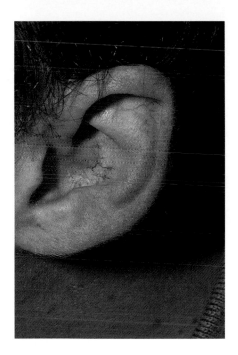

Figure 9.30 Ataxia-telangiectasia: within the pinna telangiectases are seen. Same patient as shown in Figure 9.29. This young man was 19 years old and wheelchair bound. He required a gastrostomy to ensure adequate nutrition.

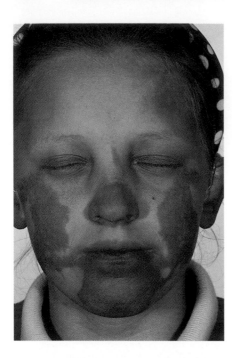

Figure 9.31 KID (keratitis, ichthyosis, deafness) syndrome: a girl of 10 years old with patterned symmetrical plaques over the cheeks and over the chin. She was deaf and partially sighted due to progressive corneal vascularization. This is a rare combination of keratitis, ichthyosis of atypical type and sensorineural deafness, which begins in infancy. Plaques appear over scalp, ears and face. A stippled skin-thickening and distorted epidermal ridge appearance over the palms and soles is striking. Hyperkeratosis over the flexures and buttocks is also seen. Inheritance is not clear-cut in this syndrome, both autosomal recessive and dominant transmission having been reported, and in fact the majority of cases described have been sporadic.

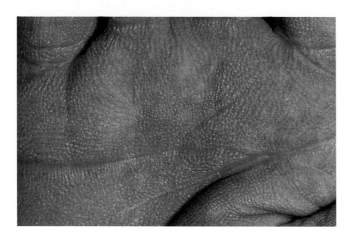

Figure 9.32 KID (keratitis, ichthyosis, deafness) syndrome: close-up of the palm of an affected adult showing striking stippled epidermal ridge appearance.

X-linked dominant

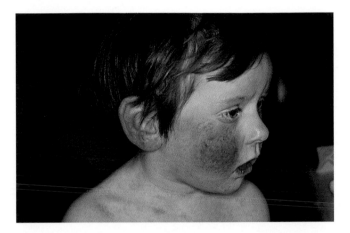

Figure 9.33 Focal dermal hypoplasia (Goltz syndrome): erythema of the cheek with depressed scar-like lesions. The child also had patches of scarring alopecia due to aplasia cutis (Chapter 5). This condition manifests with scar-like lesions, atrophy and telangiectasia, and over the face the red appearance may simulate abuse of topical corticosteroids. Hypotrichosis and short partially absent brittle nails are common. Visible subcutaneous fat may occur over posterior thighs, groin, and iliac crest areas. It is often prenatally lethal in males.

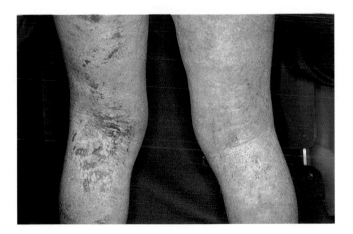

Figure 9.34 Focal dermal hypoplasia (Goltz syndrome): the same child as show in Figure 9.33 with reddish-yellow subcutaneous fat covered only by epidermis over the left popliteal fossa.

X-linked recessive

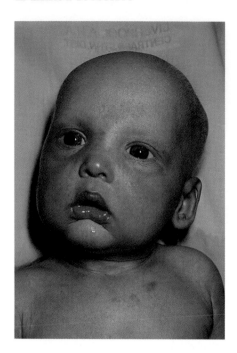

Figure 9.35 Hypohidrotic ectodermal dysplasia: a 2-month-old male showing typical facies with wrinkled periorbital skin, absent eyebrows and eyelashes, small chin, and pouting lower lip. This is usually an X-linked recessive condition in which affected individuals tend to show a similar facies, with the nose saddle-shaped with a depressed bridge, the chin small and pointed and the forehead bossed. The skin is pale, soft, thin, dry and shiny. Periorbital skin is wrinkled and hyperpigmented. Scalp hair is short, fine, usually light in colour, and scanty with eyebrows and eyelashes scanty or absent. Atopic dermatitis is often present. There is abnormal, delayed or absent dentition, affecting both deciduous and permanent teeth. The deciduous teeth tend to be widely spaced and conical. Eccrine sweat glands are absent or diminished in number and total sweating is slight. The nose is often blocked by crusts. Female carriers may show some stigmata, such as reduced sweating. In the infant, fever of obscure origin is a common presentation and an infective cause must be looked for. Avoidance of heat and excessive exercise is important but affected individuals do show an improved tolerance to environmental heat with age, relying on transepidermal perspiration.

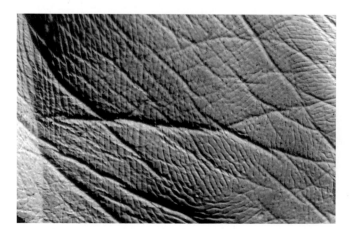

Figure 9.36 Hypohidrotic ectodermal dysplasia: a plastic imprint of the left hypothenar area of the same male as shown in Figure 9.35 at 2 months, showing flattened ridges and absent pores. With normal sweating the ridges would be elevated and pores visible.

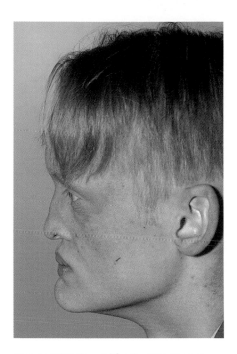

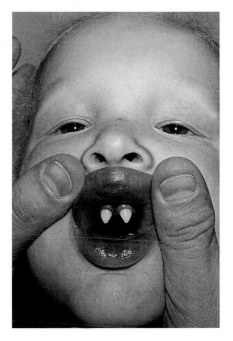

Figure 9.37 Hypohidrotic ectodermal dysplasia: the same patient as shown in Figures 9.35 and 9.36 as a young adult showing a typical profile

Figure 9.38 Hypohidrotic ectodermal dysplasia: a child of 3 years old showing characteristic pointed 'tiger' teeth.

FURTHER READING

Cnossen MH, de Goede-Bolder A, van den Broek KM, et al. A prospective 10 year follow-up study of patients with neurofibromatosis type I *Arch Dis Child* 1998; **78**: 408–12.

Giam Y-C, Khoo B-P. What syndrome is this? (Focal dermal hypoplasia (Goltz syndrome)). *Pediatr Dermatol* 1998; **15**: 399–402.

Stevens J, Lubitz L. Symptomatic zinc deficiency in breast-fed term and premature infants. *J Paediatr Child Health* 1998; **34**: 97–100.

Westerman AM, Entius MM, de Baar E, et al. Peutz-Jeghers Syndrome: 78-year follow-up of the original family. *Lancet* 1999; **353**: 1211–15.

10

Bullous Diseases, Mastocytoses and Mouth Disorders

INTRODUCTION

Impetigo including bullous impetigo, and staphylococcal scalded skin syndrome, which are more common than the other bullous conditions described in this Chapter are discussed in Chapters 1 and 3. Infants with urticaria pigmentosa are usually referred to me with unexplained itching and erythema; the typical small discrete lesions may resolve leaving hyperpigmentation which is a useful diagnostic clue.

    Examination of the mouth should be part of the general examination of a child's skin.

Bullous diseases

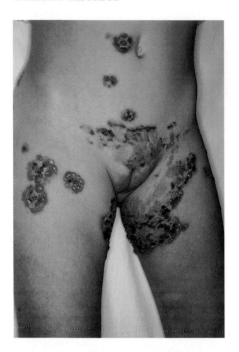

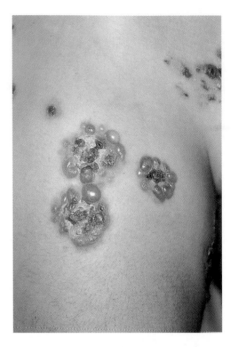

Figure 10.1 Linear IgA disease (chronic bullous disease of childhood): rosettes of blisters are particularly marked over the right thigh in this 5-year-old girl. Linear IgA disease, although a rare disorder is seen more frequently in children than either dermatitis herpetiformis or bullous pemphigoid. It is a chronic subepidermal blistering disorder characterized by the presence of IgA basement-membrane antibodies. Skin and mucosal involvement may occur. It usually begins before the age of six years and presents with tense bullae of varying sizes, some haemorrhagic. The lower half of the trunk, genitalia and lower limbs are favoured sites. Blisters often occur in ringed patterns. It responds to dapsone but this drug may not be necessary in mild cases. Conjunctival scarring may occur.

Figure 10.2 Linear IgA disease: close-up of the right thigh blister in the same child as shown in Figure 10.1.

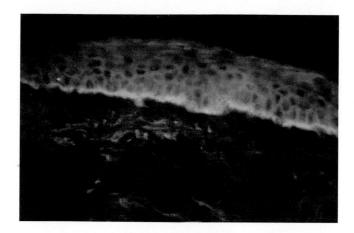

Figure 10.3 Linear IgA disease: direct immunofluorescence showing linear deposition of IgA.

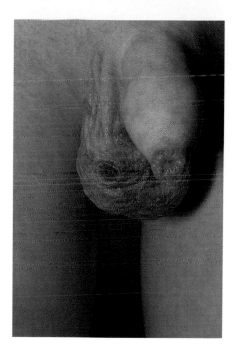

Figure 10.4 Linear IgA disease: a boy with blisters, some eroded over the scrotum which was the main site involved.

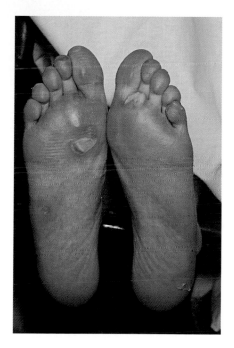

Figure 10.5 Epidermolysis bullosa (simplex – Weber-Cockayne type): a girl of 12 years old with onset of sole blisters at the age of 8 years old. She only blistered in the summer months. This dominant form of simple epidermolysis bullosa usually appears in childhood but onset may be delayed. Superficial blisters occur predominantly over the palms and soles. It is worse in warm weather and may be associated with hyperhidrosis in affected areas.

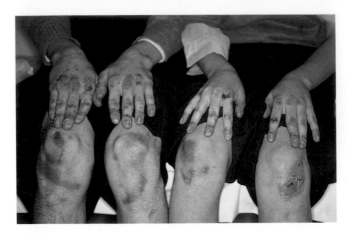

Figure 10.6 Epidermolysis bullosa (dystrophic-autosomal dominant type): brothers aged 12 and 15 years old with scarring over hands and knees following blistering. This dominant form of epidermolysis bullosa is not as severe as the recessive forms but still leaves scarring because skin separation occurs below the epidermis.

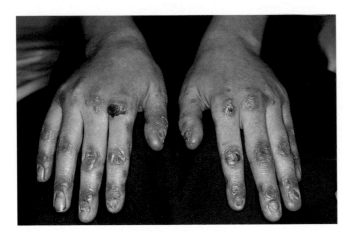

Figure 10.7 Epidermolysis bullosa (dystrophic-autosomal dominant type): a boy of 12 years old (see Figure 10.6) showing close-up of hands with scarring, erosions and dystrophic nails.

Mastocytoses

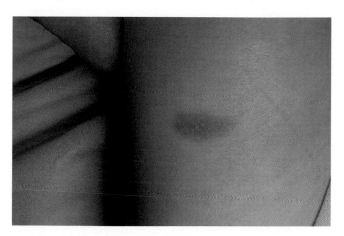

Figure 10.8 Mast cell naevus: an 8-month-old infant with a thigh lesion which appeared at 2 weeks and showed some wealing on rubbing. Mastocytoses are uncommon conditions in which there are accumulations of mast cells in the skin. Occasionally, there may be involvement of other tissues, notably bone. A *mast cell naevus* appears in infants or young children as a brownish patch or nodule which may blister at times. Sometimes, a few such naevi are present. Lesions resolve over a period of years.

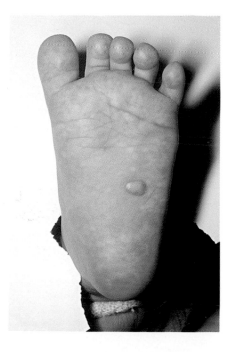

Figure 10.9 Mast cell naevus: a 7-month-old infant with a nodule over the sole.

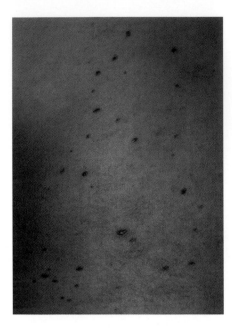

Figure 10.10 Urticaria pigmentosa: a 17-month-old infant with multiple small brownish-red papules over the back. Urticaria pigmentosa is the most common type of mast cell disease. Lesions appear in the first nine months of life. The typical lesion is a small, brown–red macule or papule which blanches on pressure or urticates after rubbing. Dermographism can commonly be elicited. Symptoms may be absent or there may be itching or flushing. Long-standing lesions show pigmentation. Oral antihistamines control symptoms and in more severe cases oral sodium cromoglycate which blocks mast cell degranulation, is also useful. The tendency is for resolution to occur but this may take many years. In most children no family history of the condition is obtained.

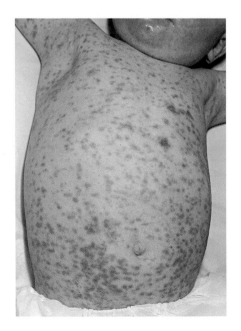

Figure 10.11 Urticaria pigmentosa: a 14-month-old infant with maculopapular orangish-red lesions. The condition appeared at 2 months of age.

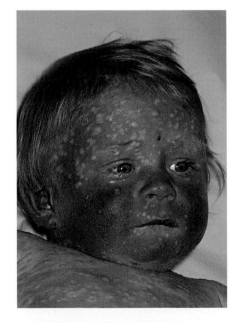

Figure 10.12 Urticaria pigmentosa: a 9-month-old boy who had widespread severe disease and was subject to flushing attacks due to histamine release.

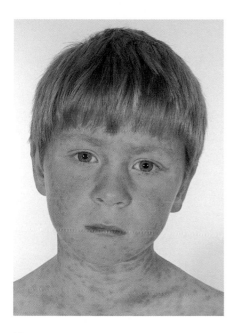

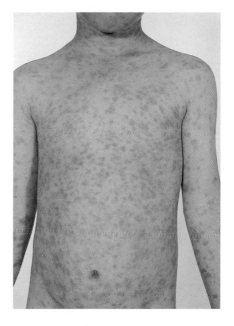

Figure 10.13 Urticaria pigmentosa: the same boy as shown in Figure 10.12 at 5 years old, much improved.

Figure 10.14 Urticaria pigmentosa: the same boy as shown in Figures 10.12 and 10.13 at 5 years showing residual macular hyperpigmentation.

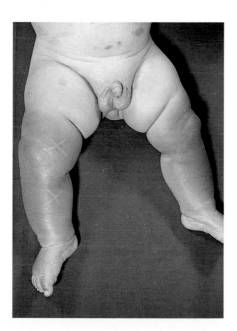

Figure 10.15 Diffuse cutaneous mastocytosis: induration and swelling of the lower limbs and dermographism is also demonstrated. In the rare diffuse cutaneous mastocytosis there is leathery skin induration: this form of mastocytosis is more likely to be associated with systemic involvement.

Mouth disorders

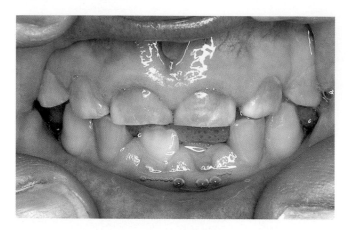

Figure 10.16 Tetracycline-stained teeth: yellowish-brown discoloration of deciduous teeth is shown. Tetracyclines should be avoided in pregnancy and also in children up to the age of 12 years old because of possible permanent yellowish-brown staining of deciduous or permanent teeth.

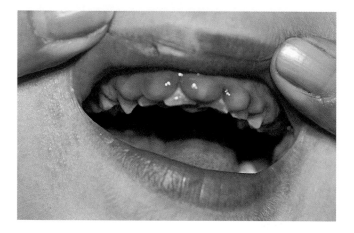

Figure 10.17 Gum hypertrophy: this was due to cyclosporin in this child, but phenytoin may also cause such hypertrophy.

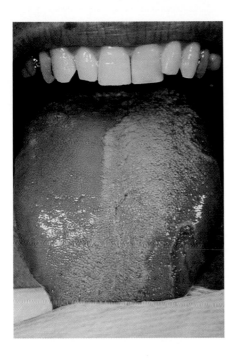

Figure 10.18 Geographic tongue (erythema migrans): dorsum of tongue showing multiple smooth red areas outlined by a white, slightly elevated margin. Map-like red areas occur with patterns changing from day to day. The tongue may be sore. Configuration of patches, which form by desquamation of filiform papillae, is constantly changing.

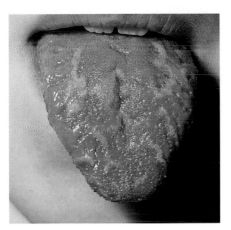

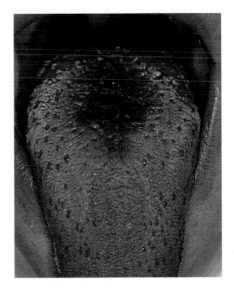

Figure 10.19 Scrotal (fissured) and geographic tongue: a 10-year-old boy showing both a scrotal and geographic appearance of the tongue. Note the white elevated margin outlining the smooth migratory patches of erythema migrans. Scrotal tongue is a developmental defect which in mild form is common. It may present in infancy. Clinically there is a deep longitudinal groove with more or less deep radiating grooves dividing the tongue into various configurations.

Figure 10.20 Black hairy tongue: a girl of 4 years old with black tongue. The condition resolved spontaneously but took more than a year to do so. This is rare in childhood. It follows a rapid proliferation of filiform papillae but the cause is unknown. This girl was well and there was no history of antibiotic ingestion.

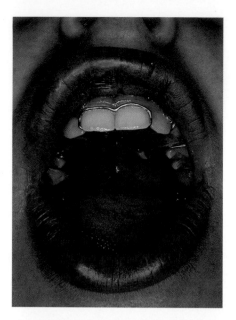

Figure 10.21 Chronic lip swelling: a girl of 11 years old with chronically swollen lips. She also showed thickening and folding of the buccal mucosa and gastrointestinal investigation revealed Crohn's disease. *Chronic lip swelling* may be post-traumatic or due to conditions such as lymphangioma, haemangioma, Crohn's disease or granulomatous cheilitis of unknown cause.

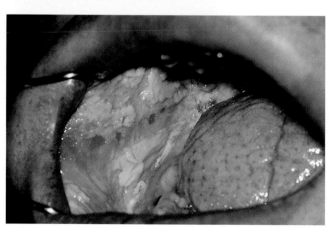

Figure 10.22 White sponge naevus: spongy patches over the buccal mucosa are shown. This rare condition is a benign epithelial irregularity that is autosomal dominant. Lesions may be present at birth and the oral mucosa is affected. They are white, thickened, folded and feel soft and spongy. Much of the buccal mucosa may be affected. Similar changes may occur in the anal canal or vulva. Antimicrobial therapy may clear lesions. Family history and examination will usually easily distinguish the mouth condition from candidosis or lichen planus.

FURTHER READING

Kettelhut BV, Metcalfe DD. Pediatric mastocytosis. *J Invest Dermatol* 1991; **96**: 15s–18s.

11

Acne, Trauma, Light Eruptions and Pigmentation Disorders

CONTENTS

INTRODUCTION

In adolescence some degree of acne is common and may have a profound effect on the quality of young life; it requires careful assessment and understanding in management. Treatment even for mild early acne is beneficial and in an early phase will generally be topical only. Steroid-induced acne may very occasionally be seen in children treated with inhaled or nasal corticosteroids: other dose-related systemic adverse effects of such preparations, including adrenal suppression, may also occur. Sunburn (acute solar dermatitis) will not usually be a reason for referral to me but unsightly actinic lentigines following sunburn are commonly seen as an incidental finding. Adequate skin protection on bright blue sky days is essential, particularly for babies, children and fair-skinned individuals. Staying in the shade especially between 11 am and 3 pm is important in sunny weather.

Acne

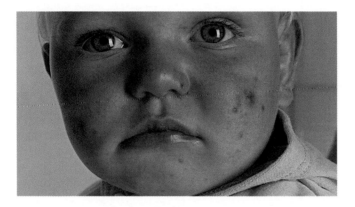

Figure 11.1 Infantile acne: inflammatory lesions over the cheek which began at 3 months of age. Infantile acne appears between the age of 3 months and 5 years and in the great majority of cases there is no evidence of endocrine disorder. Papules, pustules, nodules and cysts occur and there may be comedones (blackheads). Most cases do improve within a few years. Topical applications and if severe, oral erythromycin, can be prescribed.

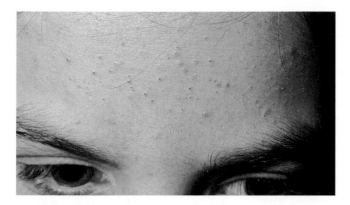

Figure 11.2 Acne vulgaris: a 12-year-old with comedones over the forehead. Acne vulgaris is so common in its mild form between the ages of 14 and 19 years that it may be considered physiological. However, it can be severe and produce both physical and mental discomfort, severely affecting the quality of life. In acne there is increased sebum production, comedogenesis, microbial colonization of pilosebaceous ducts and inflammation. Washing of the face is to be encouraged. Topical treatments include benzoyl peroxide and topical retinoids. Oral tetracyclines are first-line antibiotic therapy. The retinoid, isotretinoin, given orally, has an important place in the treatment of severe unresponsive acne but careful monitoring is essential for this teratogenic drug.

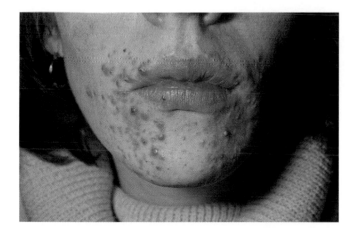

Figure 11.3 Acne vulgaris: a 17-year-old with pustular acne over and around the chin.

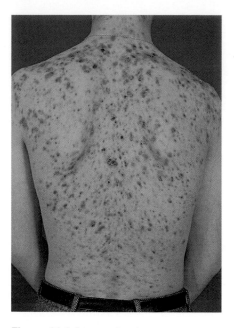

Figure 11.4 Acne vulgaris: severe, extensive, inflammatory lesions and scarring over the back.

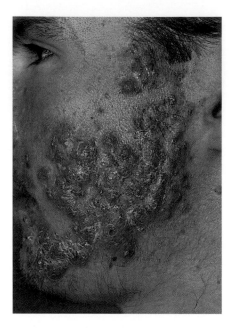

Figure 11.5 Acne vulgaris: severe, conglobate acne over the cheek. He had received topical medications and many oral antibiotics without significant improvement but did well with oral isotretinoin.

Trauma

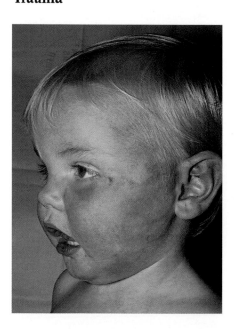

Figure 11.6 Non-accidental injury: bruising and swelling over the face. Non-accidental injury may be visible in the skin as bruising, abrasions, burns, ulceration or hair loss and it is essential to notice any unusual signs of trauma when examining a child's skin. When non-accidental injury is suspected, a child should be fully examined with a nurse present and preferably a parent also. Relevant findings should be documented with drawings and/or photographs. The child should generally be admitted under the care of a Consultant Paediatrician experienced in child abuse. *Sexual abuse* is a diagnosis that should be made with great care. It may present with allegations by the child or an adult, injuries to genitalia or anus or suspicious features such as unexplained recurrent urinary infections.

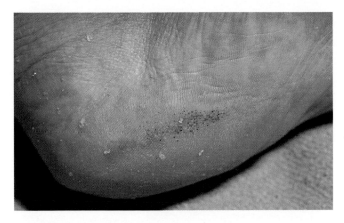

Figure 11.7 Black heel syndrome: close-up of a heel showing typical small, linear, black specks. This is a relatively common asymptomatic condition of the sole, usually bilateral and occurring in athletic adolescents. Dermal papillary capillaries are ruptured by the shearing action of the foot in shoes (often 'trainers') associated with sports such as football, cricket and basketball. It is usually noted early in the playing season and hardness of the ground seems relevant. Lesions can be mistaken for plantar warts or even malignant melanoma but the classical appearance, symmetry, bilaterality and sport history should prevent misdiagnosis.

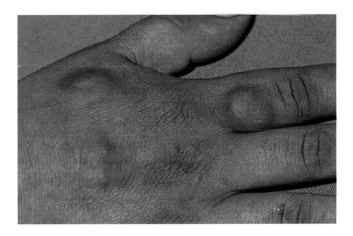

**Figure 11.8
Callosities:** a 10-year-old boy with hand callosities due to a biting habit.

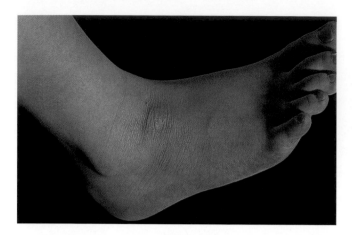

Figure 11.9 Callosity: a 6-year-old with typical *talar callosity*. This is a common, usually unrecognized lesion. Often bilateral and symmetrical, it occurs over the anterolateral aspect of the ankle (anteromedial to the lateral malleolus). Unless such a callosity is very prominent, which is uncommon, no treatment is required.

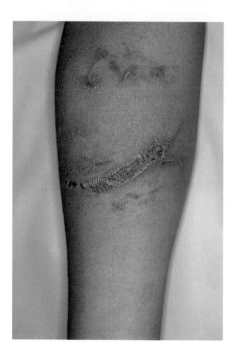

Figure 11.10 Jelly fish sting: healing lesions over the forearm, 9 days after the sting was acquired while swimming in the South of France. Skin reactions can sometimes be severe, including urticaria and ulceration. Linear painful blistering should be treated as an emergency by pouring vinegar on to the sting area and removing any attached tentacles *carefully* (to prevent further venom discharge from nematocysts) and as quickly as possible. Cold packs also provide relief. The girl shown developed acute blisters and a swollen arm but was otherwise well.

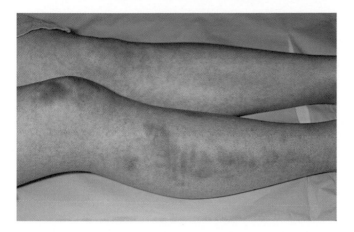

Figure 11.11 Dermatitis artefacta: a female teenager with recurrent bruising over her right knee and her right lower leg only. Dermatitis artefacta should be considered when a young person, usually female, presents with a bizarre skin eruption involving skin damage. This deliberate self-mutilation presents as ulceration, excoriations or purpura – bizarre in appearance but invariably accessible to self-infliction. Characteristically, lesions heal rapidly if occluded, only to recur with further exposure. It tends to occur in rather dull and unsophisticated children as a form of attention-seeking or protest. Usually a histrionic gesture, most cases have no significance beyond a limited nuisance value. Management includes listening carefully to the history of the appearance of the lesions and although you may take a parent into your confidence (who may not agree with your diagnosis, however!), it is generally inadvisable to directly accuse the patient of deliberately producing the lesions; he/she will not attend for follow-up if you do. Rarely, early schizophrenia may present in this way in the adolescent.

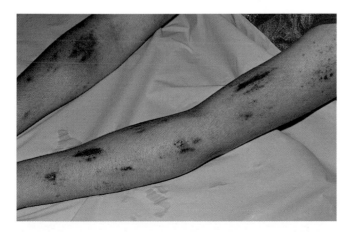

Figure 11.12 Dermatitis artefacta: bizarre, scratched excoriated lesions over the upper limbs. Similar scanty lesions were visible over the face. She had seen consultants of various disciplines with recurrent bruising inferior to the eye, also self-inflicted.

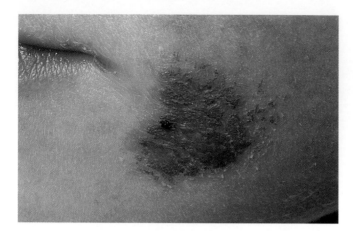

Figure 11.13
Dermatitis artefacta:
a girl of 10 years old
with an abrasion, self-
inflicted, adjacent to
the mouth.

Light eruptions

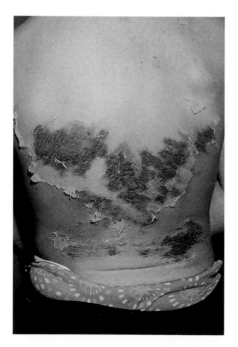

**Figure 11.14 Sunburn (acute solar
dermatitis):** skin peeling over the back
following sunburn in a 4-year-old. Calamine
lotion and mildly potent topical
corticosteroids should be applied in severe
acute sunburn. Proper preventive measures
such as cover up with loose cool clothing,
hats and sunscreen lotions of SPF 15 and
above, are most important, particularly for
infants and the fair-skinned.

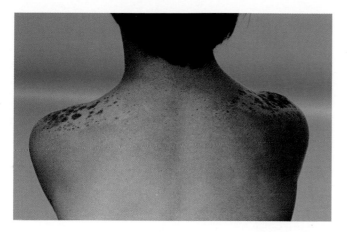

Figure 11.15 Actinic lentigo: this 9-year-old boy had repeated unprotected shoulder exposure when on holiday in Uganda. He shows hypopigmentation and pigmented macules. Such acutely sun-damaged skin may be more likely to develop malignant melanoma at a later date and adequate sun protection is a parental responsibility.

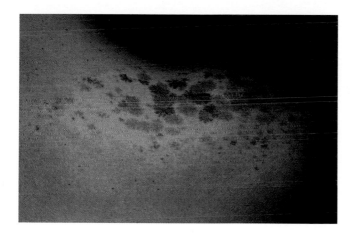

Figure 11.16 Actinic lentigo: close-up of the shoulder of same boy as in Figure 11.15, showing bizarre unsightly pigmented lesions.

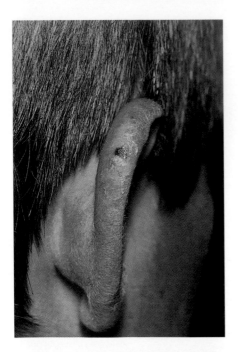

Figure 11.17 Juvenile spring eruption: a boy of 11 years old showing healing area of the helix where blistering had been present. This is not an uncommon condition manifested by small blisters, which tends to occur in boys particularly in the springtime over the light-exposed helices. It usually occurs without skin involvement elsewhere. However, it may also occur as part of *polymorphic light eruption* which is a common non-scarring entity mostly seen in young women rather than children, who show sun-induced itchy erythematous symmetrical papules over exposed areas.

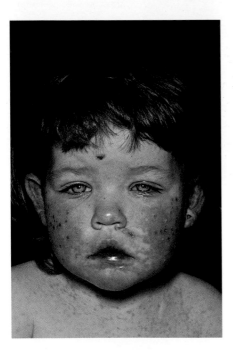

Figure 11.18 Actinic prurigo: a 2-year-old girl with excoriated papules over her cheeks. She was tearful because she also had measles. Actinic prurigo is an uncommon childhood onset eruption to which ultraviolet light A and B may contribute. It is more common in females, and worse in summer. Persistent irritant papules, often excoriated and exudative, occur not only on exposed areas but often also on covered areas such as sacrum and buttocks. Flat superficial scars may occur over face and forehead. Advice on suitable protective clothing, restriction of ultraviolet light exposure, and use of sun-screening agents with a high sun protection factor (SPF) is needed. Prognosis varies but many do clear after a few years.

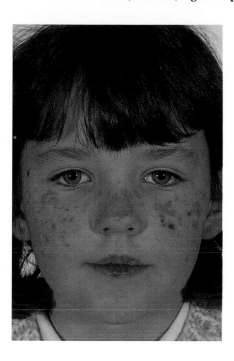

Figure 11.19 Actinic prurigo: the same girl as shown in Figure 11.18 a few years later, still developing lesions over the cheeks.

Pigmentation disorders

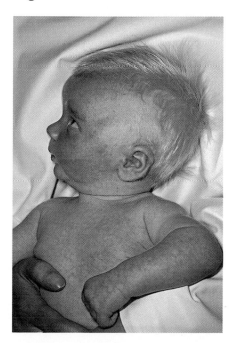

Figure 11.20 Oculocutaneous albinism: an infant with silvery white hair who has tyrosinase-positive albinism. His hair will tend to darken with age and he may show some tanning ability. Oculocutaneous albinism results from failure of melanocytes in skin, hair and eye to synthesize normal amounts of melanin. The condition is inherited as an autosomal recessive trait. The skin colour is light and the hair often whitish-yellow. The skin is very sensitive to solar radiation with the common appearance in time of solar keratoses and sometimes skin carcinoma. There is photophobia, reduced visual acuity and nystagmus. There are tyrosinase-negative and tyrosinase-positive types. From a clinical aspect, in the positive type, some pigment is formed, and such patients have the ability to tan and visual acuity may improve with age. Restriction of ultraviolet light exposure and the use of a high SPF sunscreen are essential.

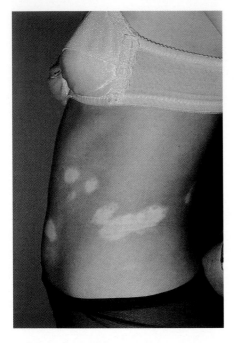

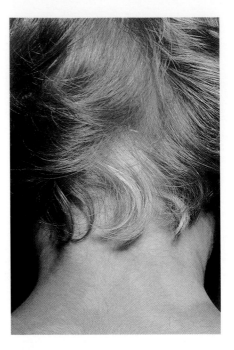

Figure 11.21 Vitiligo: unilateral, localized, segmental patchy loss of pigment in a 12-year-old girl. A common disorder said to occur in 1% of the world population. It develops before the age of 20 years in 50% of cases. There may be a positive family history. There is absence of melanocytes and melanin in the affected skin. It is usually symmetrical but vitiligo may be unilateral, and a segmental distribution is seen more commonly in children than in adults. Cosmetic camouflage, if required, and sun protection, are important.

Figure 11.22 Vitiligo: a boy with vitiligo affecting hair over the posterior of the scalp. Skin below the neck also shows some pigment loss.

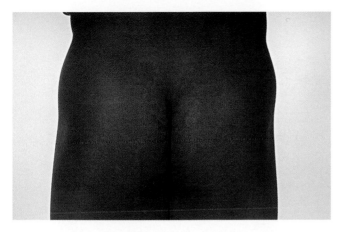

Figure 11.23 Idiopathic guttate hypomelanosis: a Nigerian boy of 10 years old with small, hypopigmented macules over the buttocks. This condition in which 2–6 mm sized white macules appear can be mistaken for vitiligo but some pigment granules are present on histology. It can also be mistaken for *pityriasis versicolor* (Chapter 3). Although it is usually over sun-exposed areas in white people, non-actinic lesions are seen in black people.

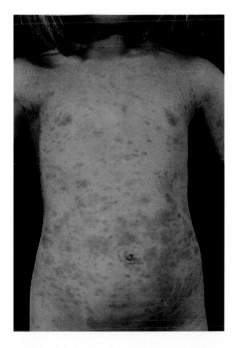

Figure 11.24 Erythema dyschromicum perstans (ashy dermatosis): widespread hyperpigmented macules of varying size are visible in this white caucasian child. This uncommon chronic condition was first described in 1957 in El Salvador. Widespread asymptomatic or slightly irritant slate grey macules or plaques appear over trunk and limbs and active lesions may show a raised edge. It tends to resolve in time. I have not seen it in children under seven years of age.

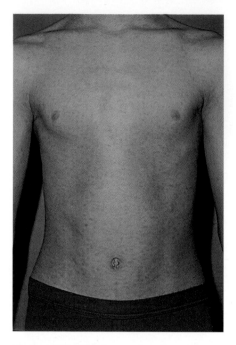

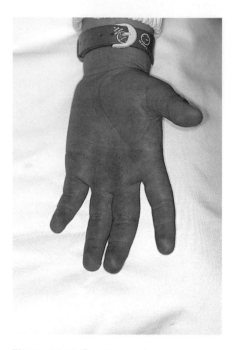

Figure 11.25 Erythema dyschromicum perstans (ashy dermatosis): a 13-year-old dark-skinned boy with patchy macular hyperpigmentation over the trunk.

Figure 11.26 Carotenaemia: orange palm in a fit female teenager who was unaware that her palm and sole skin colour was different from that of her peers. Carotene contributes to the colour of normal skin. In the presence of excessive blood-carotene levels palms and soles will show a yellow–orange discoloration. Carotenaemia is usually of no significance although it may indicate excessive intake of oranges, carrots or tomatoes. It may sometimes indicate an inborn metabolic abnormality, or be seen in diabetes or hypothyroidism.

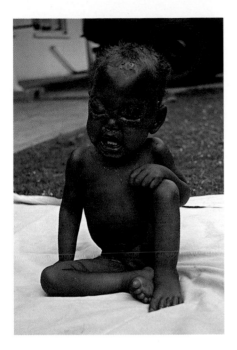

Figure 11.27 Kwashiorkor: a 2-year-old child with ulcerated skin over the face. Kwashiorkor is a common problem in children worldwide but is also seen infrequently in developed countries. It is associated with severe protein malnutrition and relative carbohydrate excess. It mostly affects children from 4 months to 4 years of age and failure to thrive is evident. Pitting oedema, usually of the lower limbs, is present. Hyperpigmented scaly plaques are especially prominent on the limbs and leave hypopigmented areas on peeling. Diffuse hair loss, and secondary bacterial infection also occur. Correction of the underlying malnutrition is the main priority with skimmed milk most useful. *Marasmus* is, like kwashiorkor, a form of protein energy malnutrition, but it results from prolonged protein and calorie starvation; it is unassociated with peripheral oedema.

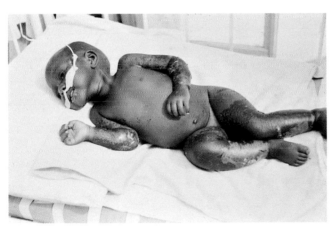

Figure 11.28 Kwashiorkor an 18-month-old infant from the Gambia with hyperpigmented plaques over the limbs and some hypopigmented areas.

FURTHER READING

Clark SM, Cunliffe WJ, Katsambas AD. Childhood/adolescent acne: a review of aetiology and management. *Curr Pediatr* 1999; **9**: 1–6.

Grabczynska SA, McGregor JM, Kondeatis E, et al. Actinic prurigo and polymorphic light eruption: common pathogenesis and the importance of HLA-DR4/DRB1*0407. *Br J Dermatol* 1999; **140**: 232–36.

Jain AM. Emergency department evaluation of child abuse. *Emerg Med Clin North Am* 1999; **17**: 575–93.

Index